Maria Emmerich
& Craig Emmerich

the Protein-Sparing Modified Fast Method

Over **120** Recipes to Accelerate
Weight Loss & **Improve Healing**

Victory Belt Publishing Inc.

Las Vegas

First published in 2022 by Victory Belt Publishing Inc.

ISBN-13: 978-1-628601-30-5

Cover and interior design and illustrations by Yordan Terziev and Boryana Yordanova

Printed in Canada

TC 0222

— table of contents —

Introduction

What Is Protein-Sparing Modified Fasting? / 7

Popular Types of Fasting / 8

Why the PSMF Method Works / 24

Starvation Mode Debunked / 35

Implementing the PSMF Method / 40

Recipes

Chapter 1: Breakfast / 52

Chapter 2: Main Dishes

Beef & Pork / 90

Poultry / 118

Seafood / 158

Chapter 3: Sides & Snacks / 208

Chapter 4: Desserts & Sweet Treats / 230

Chapter 5: Sauces & Basics / 258

Meal Plans

3 PSMF Days a Week / 278

2 PSMF Days a Week / 282

Recipe Index / 284   Allergen Index / 288

General Index / 290   More from Maria Emmerich / 302

Introduction

The obesity epidemic is growing rapidly. In 2020, the adult obesity rate in the United States hit an all-time high of 42.4 percent, which represented a 26 percent increase since 2008.[1] This is the first time the rate in any country has surpassed 40 percent. With obesity being one of the top drivers of disease, this crisis has led to type 2 diabetes, high blood pressure, reduced immune function, and many other poor health outcomes. Obesity results in increases in all of these health conditions. From 2000 to 2018, the U.S. saw the number of people diagnosed with type 2 diabetes rise from 11 million to 25 million people. That's an increase of 227 percent![2]

Studies have estimated that the healthcare costs for obesity-related illness in America were $147 billion in the year 2006.[3] That cost is only going up. Based on the 26 percent increase in obesity rates since 2008 cited above, we could be spending $185 billion or more annually on obesity-related healthcare costs today. That is about $560 a year for every person in the country, or $2,240 a year per household in obesity-related expenses. This is not sustainable. Is it any wonder that healthcare costs in the U.S. are so high compared to other countries?

The good news is that obesity is reversible! Unlike our current lack of ability to prevent cancer or other health issues, we can reverse obesity through diet and lifestyle changes. And it doesn't have to be difficult; you don't have to eat kale all day long and kill yourself in the gym for two hours every day. Weight loss is 90 percent or more about diet, and getting your macronutrients (protein, fat, and

---

[1] Centers for Disease Control and Prevention website, accessed August 6, 2021, www.cdc.gov/obesity/data/adult.html.

[2] Centers for Disease Control and Prevention website, accessed August 6, 2021, www.cdc.gov/diabetes/data/index.html.

[3] E. A. Finkelstein et al., "Annual Medical Spending Attributable to Obesity: Payer- and Service-Specific Estimates," *Health Affairs* 28, no. 5 (2009): 822–831.

carbohydrate) right will be the most significant factor in reversing obesity.

But that's not it—there is even better news! If you get the macros right and eat the foods that give you the highest satiety per calorie, you will feel full on far fewer calories, and weight loss will become easy. That is the power of protein-sparing modified fasting. It is excellent for breaking a stall and speeding up fat loss. It is a helpful tool for anyone who has undergone bariatric surgery or is trying to quickly reverse insulin resistance or other health issues—even bodybuilders looking to cut before a competition.

This book discusses what protein-sparing modified fasting is, its benefits compared to other types of fasting, and when and how often to do it. There are also many great recipes and meal plans to make this way of eating easy to implement.

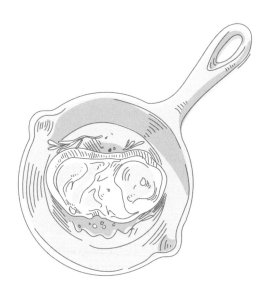

What Is Protein-Sparing Modified Fasting?

Protein-sparing modified fasting (PSMF) was first described by George Blackburn in the 1970s as a rapid weight-loss option for people with severe obesity. It is a pattern of ketogenic eating that allows you to enjoy many benefits of fasting, such as weight loss and improved insulin sensitivity, without suffering the adverse effects that you would get from other types of fasting, chief among which is the loss of lean body mass. On an extended fast, for example, you lose about one-third of a pound of lean mass each day,[4] which is not a good thing. You not only want to preserve your lean mass; you also want to build it. The "protein-sparing" part is there to assure you that this type of fasting does just that.

A ketogenic diet, where you lower your carbohydrate intake enough to force your body to use fat rather than glucose as its primary fuel, has been shown to have many health and weight-loss benefits. You see, glucose (from carbohydrates) takes priority over fat as a fuel, so your body burns any carbs you eat first, before burning fat. Therefore, when you lower the carbs in the diet, your body needs to access stored fat for fuel. This is known as becoming fat-adapted or keto-adapted.

PSMF follows the principles of ketogenic eating. That is to say, you keep carbs to a minimum, and you hit your protein goal for the day to get enough amino acids to build and repair muscle and tissues. However, with fat loss being one of the primary goals, PSMF reduces fat even more—down to a bare minimum of 20 to 30 grams daily—to ensure that your hormones remain happy and to facilitate the absorption of the fat-soluble vitamins A, D, E, and K.

As you can see, PSMF can be a powerful tool that helps you achieve rapid fat loss while keeping you healthy and strong.

---

[4]O. E. Owen et al., "Protein, Fat, and Carbohydrate Requirements during Starvation and Cataplerosis," *American Journal of Clinical Nutrition* 68, no. 1 (1998): 12–34.

Popular
Types of Fasting

The word *fasting* has received a lot of attention lately, perhaps because it seems like a quick way to lose weight. Though there are many ways to incorporate fasting into your life, you want to choose the right type of fasting to reach your goals without compromising your long-term health. Unfortunately, some types of fasting can be detrimental.

Before we get into PSMF, let's examine four other popular types of fasting, commonly used to break a stall or accelerate weight loss, as well as the effects each of them has on your health and body composition.

Fat Fasting

Fat fasting is popular in some keto communities as a way to break a stall or speed up weight loss. On a fat fast, you eat nothing but fat—coffee loaded with butter or oil, fat bombs, and other pure fats—with little to no carbs or protein.

Fat fasting is something people made up with the idea that the body can't store fat if insulin is low. Because fat consumption raises insulin only a small amount, eating only fat wouldn't raise insulin, so it wouldn't make you gain weight. But as you will see, this isn't true. Your body can store dietary fat even if you're eating only fat. It has to; if it didn't, your triglycerides (fat in the blood) would go through the roof. If you can't store the fat in your fat cells, there is no other place for it to go!

Sadly, fat fasting is a terrible strategy for getting healthy and losing weight. Here are some of the issues.

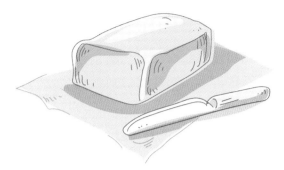

Excess dietary fat prevents fat loss

When doing a fat fast, all of the fat you eat will go into storage in your fat cells. That is the only place it can go. This isn't what you want if your goal is fat loss. The scale can and will show a drop in weight when you lose muscle mass, but this is not a good thing. Muscle is precious, and your body can't make muscle from dietary fat alone. Only amino acids in the diet plus strength training build muscle. Also, there are cells that can only run on glucose, such as red blood cells and brain neurons. If you are not eating any carbs or protein, your body can only make glucose by turning your own protein (muscle) into glucose. This and all of the daily protein needs (amino acids) to build and repair skin and other tissues require that the body cannibalize its own protein to supply what it needs.

This results in a loss of muscle or lean mass, which nobody wants. The loss of lean mass lowers your basal metabolic rate (BMR) because you have less muscle using energy all day long. With a lower BMR, you will have to eat less just to maintain your weight.

There is a lot of talk about protein in the ketogenic community. Worries about "too much protein turning into glucose" are a myth that we discuss in our book *Keto*. Getting sufficient amounts of protein is especially important for long-term health and quality of life. Maintaining lean mass as you age is critical. You don't want to be frail and immobile when you are older. And the older you get, the more protein you need (see the egg fasting section).

Focusing only on insulin has a few issues. Many keto experts insist that if insulin doesn't rise, you won't gain weight, and you will lose body fat. But there is a fundamental problem with this concept: you can—and will—gain weight if you eat enough low-insulin foods, even pure fat.

If the goal is fat loss, flooding your system with fat will achieve the opposite effect. Human biology dictates that dietary fat be stored in the fat cells once digested; that is the only place for it to go!

Let's take a look at fatty acid metabolism to see where dietary fat goes, even if you're eating only fat.

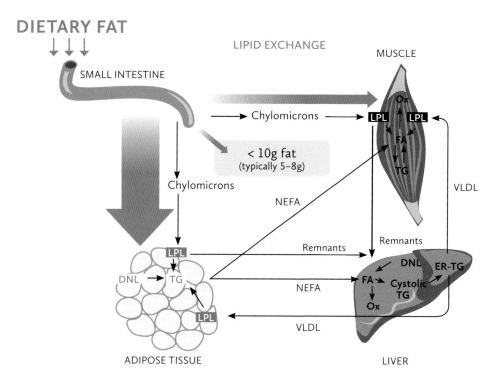

Some keto "gurus" say that fat goes right through you, but this just doesn't make sense from a biological or an evolutionary perspective. Calories were precious back in the hunter-gatherer days. If the body just dumped fat when a person ate a lot of it in the summer from the animals they hunted, they would never have made it through the lean winter months. And if you flushed large amounts of fat through your colon (more than 10 grams per day), you would live on the toilet. Remember the fat substitute Olestra and the infamous potato chips it was used in? The manufacturer had to put a label on them warning of anal leakage from an extra 10 to 20 grams of fat going through the stool.

The fact is that almost all of the fat you consume ends up in your bloodstream inside chylomicrons, tiny particles that transport dietary lipids from the intestines. Studies have shown that varying the amount of dietary fat from 93 grams to 168 grams a day resulted in no change in the amount of fat in the stool, which in this study was always less than 10 grams a day.[5] It was constant and, on average, about 8 grams a day. Where does the rest go? It gets absorbed into the body, of course. And once in the bloodstream, it can go only two places: to the cells to be burned as fuel or to adipose tissue (fat storage). And studies have shown that most of the fat goes to fat storage before being used as fuel.[6] Eating fat will quickly shut

---

[5] J. H. Cummings et al., "Influence of Diets High and Low in Animal Fat on Bowel Habit, Gastrointestinal Transit Time, Fecal Microflora, Bile Acid, and Fat Excretion," *Journal of Clinical Investigation* 61, no. 4 (1978): 953–963.

down lipolysis, the mobilization of fat from fat stores to be used as fuel (more on page 28), as the body does not want an oversupply of fat in the blood.

So how does fat get stored? There are a couple of mechanisms: insulin and acylation-stimulating protein (ASP).

The primary controller of the storing of fat is insulin. So, despite what proponents of fat fasting say, fat does raise insulin levels—not as much as protein or carbs do, but it does. And for most people, this rise in insulin is enough to get the fat stored in their adipose tissues (fat cells).

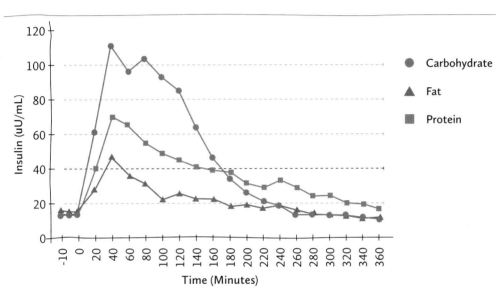

Insulin Needed to Process Macronutrients

Since the concept of fat fasting is based on misinformation about insulin, let's take a look at how this hormone works. Insulin does two things. It helps store fuels (fat and glucose) in the tissues—either muscle (glycogen) or adipocytes (fat cells). It also acts as a net to hold back fat or glucose from being released from the fat cells or liver, respectively, into the bloodstream. This makes sense because if you have a large amount of glucose or fat coming in through a meal, your body doesn't want an oversupply of fuel in your blood, so it stops adding fuel (stops lipolysis) and starts storing it to lower the blood fuel levels. The body is kind of like a car engine. You don't want to have an oversupply of fuel at any time, or you could blow up the engine. Likewise, the body likes to tightly control fuels in the blood at all times based on demand at that moment regardless of what you're doing—sitting, walking around, running a marathon, etc.

The other factor is a lesser-known process involving acylation-stimulating protein (ASP), a hormone involved in the storing of fat. This process helps put fat into storage when insulin levels aren't very high. But there is a

[6]K. N. Frayn, P. Arner, and H. Yki-Järvinen, "Fatty Acid Metabolism in Adipose Tissue, Muscle, and Liver in Health and Disease," *Essays in Biochemistry* 42 (2006): 89–103.

threshold of basal or fasting insulin to enable ASP to function properly. If you are a lean person with 10 pounds or less of excess body fat, your insulin may be low enough that this process becomes limited (fasting insulin below 2.0). If you have very low basal or fasting insulin levels and eat lots of fat, the fat has trouble getting into storage where it belongs, so it accumulates in the blood and results in very high triglycerides. Over time, if you continued eating high fat and very low protein and carbs—precisely what people do on a fat fast—your body would scramble to find places to put the fat.

Fat fasting also encourages the consumption of processed oils, such as MCT oil, in a way that is not natural. When you drink calories, it's easy to take in too many too rapidly. And when you down a large amount of fat, your system struggles to deal with the influx of energy. We don't have this scenario in nature. You don't eat pure, refined liquid fats; you eat foods like protein that contain whole, unprocessed fats—the kind you have to chew slowly and will be too full to overeat in one sitting.

How much fat you can store is dependent on your body's personal fat threshold. Your personal fat threshold is the total amount of body fat you can store in your adipose (fat) cells before they get overstuffed and inflamed. Several factors contribute to your personal fat threshold. Genetics is one of them, but the primary factor is how many fat cells you grew when you were young. You may have heard that kids can grow new fat cells. But after a certain age, no new fat cells grow; you just fill or empty the ones you have.

As an adult, you have a certain amount of body fat you can gain before metabolic dysfunction like type 2 diabetes begins to develop. When you fill up your fat cells, they become stuffed and inflamed. They then reject insulin or become insulin resistant because they don't want to burst. This is how insulin resistance begins. The body is running out of places to put fat, so fat accumulates in the blood (high triglycerides) and the liver, pancreas, and other organs. As more and more of the fat cells become stuffed and insulin resistant, the body struggles to get fuel out of the blood and into storage. So fasting or basal insulin levels rise, triglycerides and fasting glucose levels increase, blood pressure goes up, and the signs of metabolic dysfunction arise.

If you don't have many fat cells, the phenomenon described above will occur quickly, which means you have a very low personal fat threshold. If you have many fat cells, you can get much more overweight before it happens, which means you have a high personal fat threshold. This is why it is possible for a person to weigh 110 pounds and have type 2 diabetes. That person has a very low personal fat threshold. There are also people who weigh 350 pounds and do not show signs of insulin resistance because they have a very high personal fat threshold.

You are probably saying, "But I'm above my fat threshold; I still have 40 pounds to lose." In that case, you likely have enough basal insulin to store the fat eaten and for ASP to do its job. Basal insulin is the amount of insulin in the blood when fasted, or the baseline level when you're not eating. If weight loss is your goal, you don't want a bunch of fat to be stored in your fat cells. Fat is constantly going in and out of the fat cells; this is called fat flux. The fat going into the cells is dietary fat or leftover fat in the blood that the body didn't use; the fat coming out is free fatty acids that the body can use for fuel. If more fat is coming out than going in, you are in a negative fat flux. That's what you want when you're trying to lose weight. However, negative fat flux will not occur if you keep pumping dietary fat into your system and in large amounts on fat fasts.

Fat Calories Are Nutrient-Poor

You want the calories you take in to be as nutrient-dense and satisfying as possible. However, not all calories are created equal; some are more nutritive and satiating than others. A steak, for example, gives you the satisfaction of chewing as well as nutrients to build and repair your body. On the other hand, a cup of coffee loaded with butter, cream, or coconut oil gives you mostly empty calories. Just look at how many nutrients you get from eggs or beef compared to a fatty coffee for the same 400 calories.

(per 400 calories)	Butter Coffee	Eggs	Beef
Calcium (mg)	6.8	132.0	23.5
Magnesium (mg)	0.6	26.4	40.7
Phosphorus (mg)	6.8	454.0	374.5
Potassium (mg)	6.8	332.0	791.8
Iron (mg)	0.0	3.1	7.1
Zinc (mg)	0.8	2.8	9.6
Selenium (mcg)	0.3	81.3	30.4
Vitamin A (IU)	709.0	1372.8	85.6
Vitamin B6 (mg)	0.0	0.3	0.9
Vitamin B12 (mg)	0.0	2.9	4.3
Vitamin C (mg)	0.0	0.0	4.3
Vitamin D (IU)	2.9	229.7	15.0
Vitamin E (mg)	0.7	2.7	3.6
Niacin (mg)	0.0	0.2	10.3
Folate (mcg)	0.9	116.2	12.8
Protein (g)	0.2	33.0	77.0

As you can see, other than a bit of vitamin A, fatty coffee has almost zero vitamins and minerals compared to eggs and beef, which offer a lot of vitamins, minerals, and complete proteins. It's not even a close match!

Speaking of empty calories, MCT oil, which is ubiquitous in fat-fasting treats, is highly refined, loaded with empty calories, and devoid of micronutrients. Take a look at MCT oil compared to table sugar.

	Sugar (31 teaspoons)	MCT Oil (13 teaspoons)	Eggs (5¼ large)	Beef Sirloin (11 ounces)
(per 400 calories)				
Calcium (mg)	1.3	0.0	132.0	50.5
Magnesium (mg)	0.0	0.0	26.4	46.8
Phosphorus (mg)	0.0	0.0	454.0	842.0
Potassium (mg)	2.6	0.0	332.0	1197.5
Iron (mg)	0.1	0.0	3.1	9.0
Zinc (mg)	0.0	0.0	2.8	14.2
Selenium (mcg)	0.8	0.0	81.3	84.8
Vitamin A (IU)	0.0	0.0	1372.8	43.7
Vitamin B6 (mg)	0.0	0.0	0.3	2.4
Vitamin B12 (mg)	0.0	0.0	2.9	6.3
Vitamin C (mg)	0.0	0.0	0.0	7.8
Vitamin D (IU)	0.0	0.0	229.7	3.1
Vitamin E (mg)	0.0	0.0	2.7	0.9
Niacin (mg)	0.0	0.0	0.2	24.7
Folate (mcg)	0.0	0.0	116.2	15.6

Yes, this chart is correct: there are more trace vitamins and minerals in sugar than in MCT oil. You should not replace MCT oil with sugar, of course, but MCT oil is no better than sugar when it comes to nutrients. And both offer almost nothing compared to eggs and beef sirloin.

You can include some MCT oil in your diet, such as in a salad dressing or similar recipe where you want the oil to be liquid at room temperature, but you need to view it as what it is: pure energy without nutrients. In a well-formulated diet for long-term health, most of the fats should come from whole foods, not from refined oils. Therefore, it is time to ditch all of the products and treats like MCT powder and oil in coffee, butter coffee, fatty shots, fatty lattes, and fatty drinks in general. Even if you are in maintenance mode, you don't need empty calories.

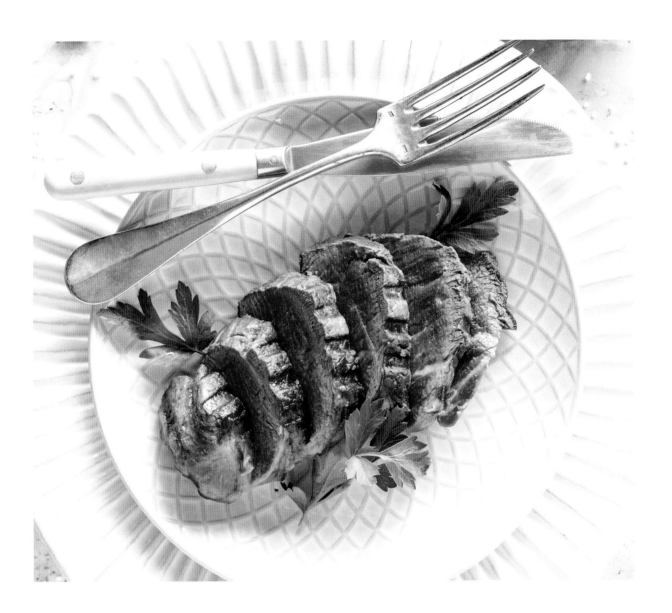

It's important to note that we are not saying to be afraid of fats. We don't fear fat; in fact, we consume lots of healthy fats from whole-food sources, such as fatty rib-eye steaks and other meats and some dairy in sauces, up to our maintenance level of fat and calories. However, when fat loss is the goal, your diet doesn't need to be high in fat. By dialing down the dietary fat, you let your body use its own stored fat for fuel.

For these two main reasons, we do not recommend fat fasting to anyone. It's a way to achieve fat loss that offers no real benefits but comes with many negatives. Instead, stick with whole foods and enjoy all of the vitamins and minerals that come with them. Eat the fats that come with your proteins, being careful not to consume them too liberally if fat loss is the goal. You will always have better long-term health by eating more nutrient-dense foods.

Egg Fasting

Just as you eat nothing but fat on a fat fast, you eat no foods other than eggs on an egg fast. Egg fasting used to be quite popular, and it's still practiced in some keto communities that believe this type of fasting will break a stall or speed up weight loss.

While eggs are a healthy food, we don't recommend egg fasting. There are a couple of issues with this type of fast.

One problem with egg fasting is that it's tough to get enough protein. You need about 0.8 times your lean mass in protein grams per day to maintain muscle and lean mass. For example, a woman, who is 5 feet 4 inches tall and weighs 150 pounds with 30 percent body fat has 105 pounds of lean mass. This means she needs a minimum of 84 grams of protein per day to maintain her lean mass. If she wants to gain muscle, she will need more. And if she is over 50, she will need even more protein due to a leucine shift. The minimum amount of the amino acid leucine required to trigger muscle protein synthesis increases as a person gets older. Considering that people who are over 50 and 60 years old need 0.9 and 1.0 times lean mass, respectively, just to maintain the lean mass, this woman would need closer to 100 to 120 grams of protein daily. This translates to about 18 large eggs. A man of typical height would have to eat even more—about 24 eggs a day!

This leads us to the other issue with egg fasting: you get really sick of eggs really quickly. Making you sick of eating eggs is probably the most effective thing egg fasting does! We love eggs, but we would be sick of them after a day or two of eating 18 to 24 eggs per day. We believe this is the case with most people who lose weight on egg fasts: they simply get sick of eggs and undereat as a result. Even if you manage to eat 8 or 9 eggs in a day—and that's a lot of eggs for one day—you are getting only about 50 grams of protein. Failure to meet your daily protein goal will result in muscle loss over time. The scale may be moving, but at the cost of your long-term health.

You need a fast that allows for a variety of tasty, protein-rich, and nutrient-dense foods—including eggs!—not a fast that makes you eat nothing but eggs only to make you sick of eating them.

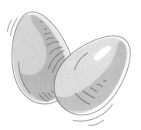

Extended Fasting

Extended fasting involves consuming little to no calories for at least 24 hours. It is quite popular in several keto communities.

Some extended-fasting practices recommend eating only every other day, while others promote eating nothing for three days or more. This may cause a drop in weight. However, as mentioned earlier, some of that loss will be muscle loss, which you do not want.

In addition, extended-fasting gurus often neglect to focus on what you should eat when not fasting. As a result, some people break their fast with unhealthy foods, such as pasta or bread, in large amounts. This has many detrimental effects. Putting your body in and out of ketosis in this way forces it into a cycle of being flooded with glucose only to run out of it and have to cannibalize its own lean mass. Studies have shown that people lose more than a pound of lean mass in the first day or two of fasting and about a quarter of a pound per day after that.[7]

Many people do extended fasting to enter a stage of autophagy, where the body takes the cells apart, removes any damage, and rebuilds new cells from what's left. This can be an effective tool for people who are very sick with illnesses such as cancer or who have significant organ damage; the body can, in some cases, turn over the bad cells and make new healthier ones. Fasting also induces apoptosis, whereby the body kills and removes damaged or bad cells that cannot be recycled. This, too, is beneficial, but it should be done only under medical supervision.

We feel that fasting gurus put way too much faith in autophagy. Autophagy is made out to be the "fountain of youth," the benefits of which can be experienced only when you eat nothing for long periods. This just isn't true. First, autophagy is happening all the time at varying levels. Yoshinori Ohsumi, who won the Nobel Prize in 2016 for his research on autophagy, estimates that, on average, we turn over all of the protein cells in our bodies in two to three months.[8] This happens without fasting! In fact, up to 20 percent of our basal metabolic rate (BMR) is from autophagy.

Guess what stimulates autophagy as much as—if not more than—fasting? Exercise and strength training! And unlike fasting, exercise and strength training help you build muscle instead of causing you to lose it.

Many research studies have shown this to be true. For example, a 2012 study found that treadmill exercise induced autophagy in the cerebral

[7]O. E. Owen, K. J. Smalley, D. A. D'Alessio, M. A. Mozzoli, and E. K. Dawson, "Protein, Fat, and Carbohydrate Requirements During Starvation: Anaplerosis and Cataplerosis," *American Journal of Clinical Nutrition* 68, no. 1 (1998): 12–34.

[8]The Nobel Prize website, accessed August 6, 2021, www.nobelprize.org/prizes/medicine/2016/ohsumi/facts/.

cortexes of adult mice.[9] Another found that exercise induced autophagy through BLC2 genes, which are a crucial regulator of exercise-induced autophagy, and that autophagy induction may contribute to the beneficial metabolic effects of exercise.[10] A 2015 study found that subjects receiving continuous glucose infusions during a 60-minute exercise session had greater autophagy signaling than those doing a 36-hour fast.[11] Another study found that the most effective strategy to activate autophagy in human skeletal muscle seemed to rely more on exercise intensity than on diet.[12]

For us, the takeaway from these studies and many others is this: we would rather eat a filet mignon for a lean protein boost and lift weights to enhance our cellular health than eat nothing for one or more days and lose muscle.

A 2021 study looked at alternate-day fasting, where one group of participants ate nothing every other day and ate 150 percent of maintenance calories on the other days. The control group did no fasting and simply ate at a 25 percent calorie deficit every day. Both groups ate the exact same number of calories each week. The striking differences in fat mass and lean mass between the two groups show how detrimental extended fasting is to body composition.[13]

A randomized controlled trial to isolate the effects of fasting and energy restriction on weight loss and metabolic health in lean adults

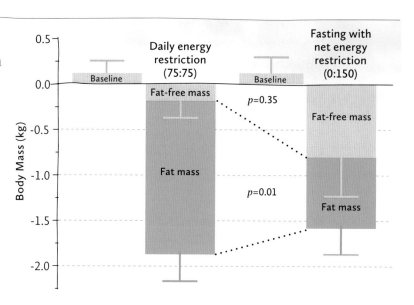

[9]C. He, R. Sumpter, Jr., and B. Levine, "Exercise Induces Autophagy in Peripheral Tissues and in the Brain," *Autophagy* 8, no. 10 (2012): 1548–1551.

[10]C. He et al., "Exercise-Induced BCL2-Regulated Autophagy Is Required for Muscle Glucose Homeostasis," *Nature* 481, no. 7382 (2012): 511–515.

[11]A. B. Moller et al., "Physical Exercise Increases Autophagic Signaling through ULK1 in Human Skeletal Muscle," *Journal of Applied Physiology* 118, no. 8 (1985): 971–979.

[12]C. Schwalm et al., "Activation of Autophagy in Human Skeletal Muscle Is Dependent on Exercise Intensity and AMPK Activation," *FASB Journal* 29, no. 8 (2015): 3515–3526.

[13]I. Templeman et al., "A Randomized Controlled Trial to Isolate the Effects of Fasting and Energy Restriction on Weight Loss and Metabolic Health in Lean Adults," *Science Translational Medicine* 16, no. 13 (2021): 598.

The participants who fasted lost over twice as much muscle mass (lean or fat-free mass) and less than half as much body fat (fat mass). They also lost less weight overall. The study looked for markers of insulin resistance and post-meal blood sugar levels and found no significant difference between the two groups.

The last thing this study looked at was markers for inflammation and autophagy. Possibly the most remarkable result is that there were no favorable changes in gene expression of inflammation and autophagy! This is in direct contrast to the message spread by proponents of extended fasting that extended fasting lowers inflammation and increases autophagy.

Another negative effect of extended fasting is a reduced frequency of bowel movements. We store toxins in our fat cells, and when we lose body fat, those toxins are released into the bloodstream. One of the primary ways the toxins get detoxed is through the stool. So what happens to all of these toxins when you aren't eating anything for multiple days and thus aren't going number two? They are reabsorbed into your body. This is not healthy and can lead to the accumulation of bad estrogens (estrogen dominance) and other toxins. Therefore, it is important to have a bowel movement every day, especially when losing body fat.

When done under medical supervision, extended fasting may be a helpful tool for someone with cancer or a serious illness who wants to accelerate the purging of unhealthy cells. However, if weight loss is your goal, extended fasting will only make you weaker with less muscle mass. And since less muscle mass means a lower BMR, you will require fewer calories just to maintain your weight. For fat loss, general health, or disease prevention, you want to eat a well-formulated ketogenic diet. Long-term fasting is neither necessary nor beneficial.

In summary, we don't recommend extended fasting for weight loss or general health. The negatives outweigh any minor benefits from autophagy. In fact, if autophagy is your goal, strength training and exercise will be more beneficial to you and your weight-loss goals.

Intermittent Fasting

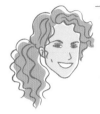

When I first heard about intermittent fasting, I remember thinking, "No, no, no, this is not good for anyone who wants to maintain muscle!" But after diving into what happens when you fast on a well-formulated keto diet, I realized that not only would you maintain muscle, but you would enjoy other benefits as well. I now work and write early in the morning in a fasted state for about three hours, and my mind has never been clearer. In this state, your ketone levels will likely be higher, which can lead to more mental clarity.

Intermittent Fasting

Increases

⬆ Leptin levels to reduce overeating

⬆ Insulin and leptin sensitivity, lowering risk of diabetes, heart disease, and cancer

⬆ Ability to become keto-adapted, turning you into a fat burner!

Decreases

⬇ Triglycerides, lowering heart disease risk

⬇ Inflammation and free radical damage

⬇ Weight gain and metabolic disease risk

Example Schedule

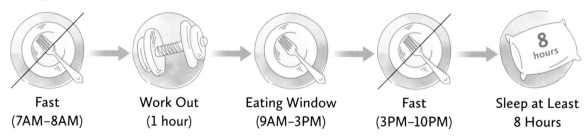

| Fast (7AM–8AM) | Work Out (1 hour) | Eating Window (9AM–3PM) | Fast (3PM–10PM) | Sleep at Least 8 Hours |

If you are pregnant or nursing or you have metabolic syndrome, don't fast. Wait until you are no longer breastfeeding or have fixed your insulin issues.

Unlike extended fasting, intermittent fasting does not require you to eat nothing at all for one or more days at a time. Instead, you restrict your daily eating to a shorter-than-typical window of time—perhaps six to eight hours. We find it to be an excellent strategy for most people.

Intermittent fasting came into our lives almost by accident. When we started eating keto, not only were we losing weight, but we were no longer "hangry." When you focus on eating nutrient-dense foods like animal protein, egg yolks, and organ meats, your cells are satiated. And when your hunger levels and cravings subside from eating a ketogenic or carnivore diet (eating no plants), intermittent fasting happens naturally.

We find it interesting that with most diets, the mental aspect, which in the case of keto is recognizing that you need to cut carbohydrates, is easy, whereas the physical part—the act of making the necessary changes—is hard. With intermittent fasting, however, it's the mental part that keeps many of our clients from even attempting it. It sounds impossible to them, so they don't even try.

We were there once, too. We like eating, and we did not relish the idea of fasting—at least we thought we didn't. However, since we were sugar burners at the time, we always wanted to eat. When you eat a high-carb diet, your body runs primarily on glucose, making you a sugar burner. Now that we are keto-adapted, we are no longer plagued by thoughts of food all day. Once you're keto-adapted, your primary fuel is fat, so you have much longer-lasting and more stable fuel for your body. Intermittent fasting comes easy once you are keto-adapted.

That being said, intermittent fasting isn't a requirement for weight loss. It's merely a pattern of eating; it's not a diet that provides a set of guidelines or rules on what to eat. You could eat poorly while practicing intermittent fasting, which would not be very helpful for your weight-loss goal or your health. Intermittent fasting is just a tool to help you get your macros right—and that is the most important thing for weight loss—by eating less often.

We recommend intermittent fasting to most people looking to lose weight. This is because intermittent fasting can be a good tool for limiting snacking and getting your macros right for fat loss. And if you start out with a keto or carnivore diet and are keto-adapted, you're not hungry all day, and this pattern of eating comes naturally to you.

Protein-Sparing Modified Fasting

Protein-sparing modified fasting (PSMF) is a great alternative to extended fasting. It provides many of the same benefits of rapid weight loss while preventing the loss of lean mass (muscle).

The PSMF method works wonderfully for the following groups:

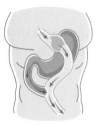

Gastric bypass patients who want to focus on real protein instead of nutrient-poor whey protein shakes

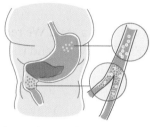

People with insulin resistance and type 2 diabetes looking to reverse insulin resistance by shrinking fat cells

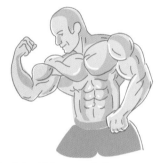

Bodybuilders and fitness competitors looking to cut (shed body fat while maintaining muscle)

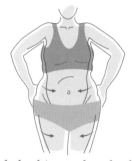

People looking to lose body fat and break weight-loss stalls

The idea behind PSMF is to reduce carbs and fat as much as possible while still hitting or even exceeding your protein goal to help with satiety. This method mimics an extended fast by forcing your body to use stored fat for fuel, thereby breaking stalls or accelerating weight loss.

However, unlike an extended fast, PSMF offers enough protein for you to feel satiated and enjoy the added benefit of the high thermic effect of protein-rich foods, which means that you effectively lose 25 to 30 percent of the calories you take in. Plus, you are eating nutrient-dense animal protein, so you are getting the vitamins and minerals your body needs. The PSMF method also provides you with enough fat—about 30 grams a day—to keep your hormones happy and to help your body absorb the fat-soluble vitamins A, D, E, and K.

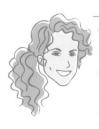

Ten years ago, I called the practice of protein-sparing modified fasting a "pure protein day." Back then, I hadn't heard of PSMF. I just knew about the thermic effect of food and how metabolism works, so I knew this method could help people lose weight faster. PSMF is becoming more well known and popular and is a great tool for improving results.

PSMF is a tool. It is something you can do occasionally to speed up fat loss or break a stall. We recommend that our clients do one to three days of PSMF in a week and then use regular fat-loss macros on the other days (our book *Keto* goes into detail about well-formulated keto macros for fat loss). It is also a good idea to do an overfeeding day during these weeks in order to shake up your metabolism (read more about the starvation mode myth on page 35 and metabolic adaptation on page 37).

It's important to note that if you are already very lean, the PSMF method probably isn't for you. This method is a tool to force the body to burn more of its own fat for fuel. So, if you don't have a lot of body fat to begin with, doing protein-sparing modified fasts will not be fun, and you don't need to do them unless you are a bodybuilder or fitness competitor looking to cut before a competition.

We find it strange that some people say the PSMF method is dangerous or unhealthy and then say that extended fasting is OK on occasion. PSMF is literally just a less-extreme extended fast. It does not lead to a loss of lean mass; it's an *improvement* on extended fasting! So, if extended fasting is OK from time to time, why would PSMF be considered dangerous?

After almost one year of intermittent fasting and many extended fasts that got me down over 30 pounds, I found you guys. I was frustrated at how stalled I was and stumbled upon PSMF.

I'm only on my third week of doing PSMF on Mondays, Wednesdays, and Fridays. I have to say (and my husband has agreed) that I am looking leaner since I started. I also feel like the little exercise I do (less than 40 minutes and not even daily) is providing more noticeable results.

Thank you, Craig and Maria, for all you do. I keep learning and improving. And best of all? I'm eating amazing food daily!

- Esther

Why
the PSMF Method Works

The PSMF method is a powerful tool for speeding up fat loss and breaking weight-loss stalls because it leverages your biology to make fat loss quick and easy. Let's take a look at some of the mechanisms and biological factors behind it.

The Thermic Effect of Food

The thermic effect of food (TEF) refers to the increase in metabolic rate that occurs after you eat. Some foods (protein) require much more energy to consume and digest than others (carbs and fat). This means that the total calories consumed will result in different amounts of effective calories in the body depending on which macronutrients were eaten:

Macronutrient	Average Thermic Effect of Food	Calories Consumed	Effective Calories
Fat	3%	100	97
Carbohydrate	8%	100	92
Protein	25%	100	75

As you can see, fat has a very low TEF (3 percent), meaning that almost all of the fat calories you consume end up in storage because fat is easy to digest and process. Carbohydrate has a higher TEF at 8 percent. But protein has the highest at 25 percent on average, over three times higher than the other macronutrients; it can be up to 30 percent depending on the source. Protein takes a lot of energy to digest and process, which means that 25 percent of its calories effectively don't count.

This chart shows how protein results in fewer effective calories in the body. The PSMF method is a powerful tool for weight loss for this reason. Not only are you significantly limiting the fuel coming in through your diet, but the protein you focus on enables you to burn more calories due to its high TEF. Together, reducing calorie intake and prioritizing protein force your body to use more stored body fat for fuel, resulting in fat loss.

Oxidative Priority

Oxidative priority is the order in which the body processes and stores fuels from the diet. Fuels with higher priority must be processed before lower-priority fuels. The body likes to have tight control over the fuels in the bloodstream at any given moment based on the current demand. If you are at rest, there are less than 100 calories of total energy in your bloodstream from glucose, fat, and ketones. When you eat a meal, an enormous amount of energy floods into your blood, so your body has to prioritize how to store it and which sources to use first to prevent an oversupply of fuel. You can die from having too much glucose, fat, or ketones in your blood.

The way the body prioritizes fuels makes a lot of sense; it does so in reverse order of storage capacity. Thus, things for which it has no storage, like alcohol, have to be burned, whereas things that are easy to store and for which it has large storage space (fat) can be stored and dealt with later.

Here is a chart showing the oxidative priority of fuels.

Oxidative Priority
How the body prioritizes fuels

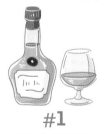

#1
ALCOHOL
Storage capacity:
0 calories

#2
EXOGENOUS KETONES
Storage capacity:
0 calories

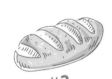

#3
CARBS
Storage capacity:
1,200–2,000 calories

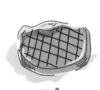

#4
PROTEIN
Storage capacity:
360 calories

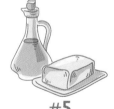

#5
FAT
Storage capacity:
almost unlimited calories

If supply (food intake) is greater than demand, lower-priority fuels get stored first.

The number one priority is alcohol because the body cannot store it. So it must burn off all alcohol before it can get to burning other fuels. This means that if you eat a meal while drinking alcohol, most of the food will be stored while your body deals with the booze. This is one reason why alcohol consumption can be detrimental to fat loss. Therefore, if fat loss is your goal, then avoiding alcohol is best. In fact, we recommend excluding it on PSMF days.

The next highest priority is exogenous ketones, such as from ketone drink supplements. We do not recommend using them in any situation other than for certain brain issues like seizures and Alzheimer's. If fat loss is your goal, adding exogenous ketones is not going to help you. Let your body make its own ketones from your fat stores.

Next are carbohydrates. The body has a moderate storage capacity for carbs in the liver and muscle, but only about 1,500 to 2,000 calories can be stored as glycogen. And the glycogen stored in muscle is locked into the muscle and really only used during intense workouts like sprints or long runs of two hours or more. A one-hour vigorous walk will likely tap little to none of this glycogen. So really, you have only your liver for storage, which can hold maybe 100 grams of glucose. Any excess beyond storage capacity or fuel needs is turned into fat and stored in fat cells.

The next priority is protein. Protein is used as a fuel only when there aren't other fuels available from the diet or the body. So, if you are very lean (and thus do not have a lot of stored fat) and eat very low fat and carbs, your body will turn protein into glucose to supply itself with fuel. But for most people, including anyone who wants to lose fat, protein is used to build and repair lean tissues. Our bodies are constantly turning over protein and need a constant supply of amino acids to fuel this turnover. Hitting your protein goal (or maybe a bit more for PSMF days) will ensure that you have enough to maintain your lean mass.

The last priority is fat. This makes sense because fat is the easiest to store, and we have almost unlimited storage space for it (some people have over a million calories stored as fat). However, dietary fat will prevent your own body fat from being used as fuel. There are only three biological pathways for dietary fat. Either it is passed right through into the stool and not absorbed, or it is digested and absorbed. If it is absorbed, it is either used as fuel for the cells or stored in your fat cells. As explained on page 9, the vast majority of the fat you eat ends up in storage. This is not what you want if fat loss is your goal.

Therefore, by focusing on protein and eliminating or limiting other fuels (alcohol, exogenous ketones, carbs, and fat) on PSMF, you force your body to use more of its stored fat as fuel. This makes PSMF a powerful and effective method for fat loss.

Did you know that it takes the average person six hours of fasting (eating nothing) to metabolize the fat in one cup of bulletproof coffee (BPC)? This is why I don't understand the recommendation to drink a BPC to "extend a fast." There are no metabolic improvements from fasting for another couple of hours that will overcome the calories in a BPC.

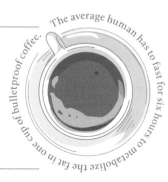

The average human has to fast for six hours to metabolize the fat in one cup of bulletproof coffee.

The Krebs Cycle

One of the concerns people have raised to us over the years is that their ketone levels go down when they eat more protein. To that we say, you don't want to chase ketones if weight loss is your goal. There is no correlation between blood ketones and weight loss. You can have very high blood ketone levels and be gaining body fat if you're drinking bulletproof coffees and eating high-fat foods.

So what is going on with ketones when you eat more protein? Here's the biology.

Energy metabolism is very complex, but let's break it down into its most basic form first. Here is an illustration of a triglyceride molecule. Notice that the free fatty acid molecules are just long chains of carbon and hydrogen molecules.

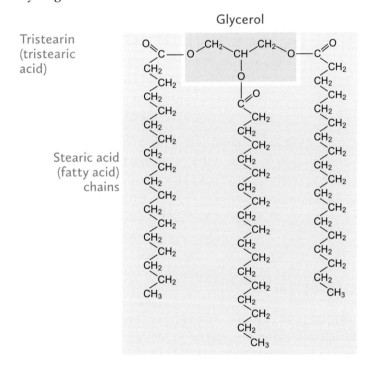

The whole cycle is known as cellular respiration. First, you breathe in oxygen, which is an O_2 molecule (two oxygen atoms linked together). The body then takes fats or carbohydrates (from the body or diet) and strips off the hydrogen ions to fuel the mitochondria, the power centers of your cells. Yes, you are a little like an electronic device getting your energy from electrons (hydrogen atoms). The carbon that remains is then attached to the oxygen molecule to create CO_2, and you breathe it out. So, with every breath, you are taking in oxygen, grabbing the leftover carbon from your food, and exhaling it as carbon dioxide. Pretty simple, right? Well, not actually.

ENERGY

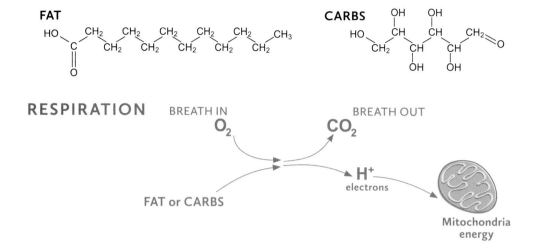

FAT

CARBS

RESPIRATION

BREATH IN O_2

BREATH OUT CO_2

H^+
electrons

FAT or CARBS

Mitochondria
energy

The citric acid cycle or Krebs cycle (also called the tricarboxylic acid cycle or TCA cycle) is the process the body uses to generate adenosine triphosphate (ATP) from carbohydrate, fat, and protein. ATP is the energy that the mitochondria use for fuel. The Krebs cycle is the primary process for turning the food you eat into energy that your cells can use to keep you alive and healthy. Let's take a deeper look at how fatty acid metabolism works in the body.

If you look at the illustration on the opposite page, you can see why they call it a cycle. It is a circular process—more on that in a minute. Before the Krebs cycle can start, the fat needs to be broken (for fatty acid metabolism) into acetyl coenzyme A (acetyl-CoA) using water and other molecules. So let's take a step back and review the entire process.

Beta-oxidation or lipolysis is the process of burning fat for fuel. The fat in your body is stored primarily as triglyceride molecules in your fat cells. A triglyceride is three free fatty acid (FFA) molecules linked together with a glycerol molecule. The first step in the beta-oxidation process is to cut the glycerol away from the fatty acids. It then goes into circulation (the bloodstream) as glycerol and three FFA molecules (FFA binds to albumin to travel in the blood, labeled NEFA on the chart on page 10). The glycerol travels to the liver. There, it is repackaged into a triglyceride molecule and sent back into fat storage inside a VLDL particle, or the liver can take three glycerol molecules to make one glucose molecule. This is called fat flux, and it is the cycle of fat going in and out of your fat cells that is happening all the time at different levels based on the current demand for fuel. (See our book *Keto* for more on fat flux.)

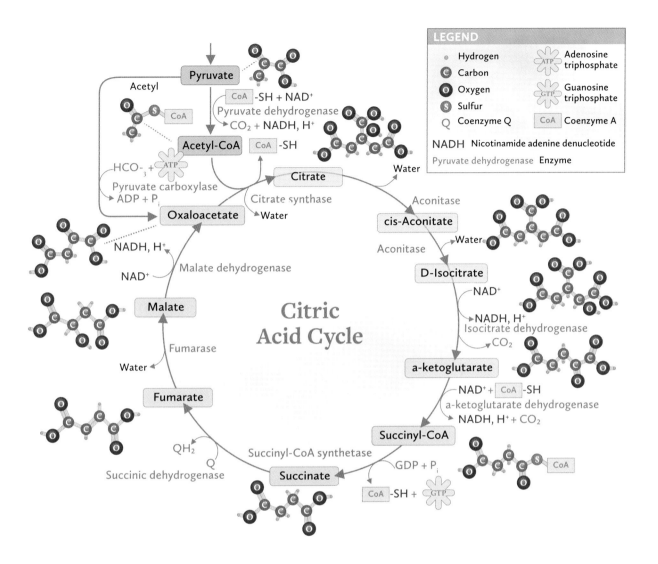

LEGEND

- · Hydrogen
- C Carbon
- O Oxygen
- S Sulfur
- Q Coenzyme Q
- ATP Adenosine triphosphate
- GTP Guanosine triphosphate
- CoA Coenzyme A

NADH Nicotinamide adenine denucleotide
Pyruvate dehydrogenase **Enzyme**

Pyruvate

Acetyl

CoA -SH + NAD⁺
Pyruvate dehydrogenase
CO_2 + NADH, H⁺

Acetyl-CoA   CoA -SH

HCO⁻₃ + ATP
Pyruvate carboxylase
ADP + P$_i$

Citrate

Water

Citrate synthase
Water

Oxaloacetate

Aconitase

cis-Aconitate

Aconitase
Water

NADH, H⁺

NAD⁺

Malate dehydrogenase

D-Isocitrate

NAD⁺

NADH, H⁺
Isocitrate dehydrogenase
CO_2

Malate

Citric Acid Cycle

a-ketoglutarate

Fumarase

NAD⁺ + CoA -SH
a-ketoglutarate dehydrogenase
NADH, H⁺ + CO_2

Water

Fumarate

Succinyl-CoA

QH₂

Q

Succinic dehydrogenase

Succinyl-CoA synthetase

Succinate

GDP + P$_i$

CoA -SH + GTP

CoA

Once the free fatty acids enter a cell, they are prepared for the Krebs cycle by being chopped into many acetyl CoAs. The main function of acetyl CoAs is to carry the acetyl group to the Krebs cycle. Thus, an acetyl group is just cut-up chunks of the FFA molecule.

The first step of the Krebs cycle is to combine the acetyl group (from the acetyl CoA) with an oxaloacetate molecule (also known as oxaloacetic acid, or OAA) to form a six-carbon citrate molecule (hence the name citric acid cycle). It then goes through a series of processes using water and other molecules going around the Krebs cycle. Every trip through this cycle generates one ATP molecule (energy for mitochondria) and two carbon dioxide molecules. But this first step is where things get interesting with respect to ketone production.

The first step in burning FFA as fuel in your cells is to combine it with an oxaloacetate molecule. Where does oxaloacetate come from? It is sourced from pyruvate, which you can think of as half of a glucose molecule. So, if you are eating a ketogenic diet, where does your body get oxaloacetate? Mostly from protein, which is turned into glucose via a process called gluconeogenesis. This is another reason not to fear gluconeogenesis, a misconception that some in the keto world promote.

But what happens if you are eating low carb *and* low protein? Your body does not have enough oxaloacetate to burn all of the fat you are eating as fuel directly. That means it now has too much fat around that it can't burn as fuel through the Krebs cycle. To keep you alive, it has to bypass the Krebs cycle and create fuel for your cells another way. It does so by turning more FFA molecules into ketone bodies (molecules of ketones) and sending them into your blood. Therefore, your blood ketone levels will rise when you are fasting, doing a fat fast, or eating a low-protein keto diet. The body doesn't have enough carbs or protein coming in, so it doesn't have enough oxaloacetate to burn fat in the Krebs cycle. Plus, some of the oxaloacetate is redirected to fuel more gluconeogenesis (GNG) to make glucose for the cells that have no mitochondria and can only run on glucose, like the brain neurons and red blood cells. This is why you lose muscle and lean mass when fasting for long periods.

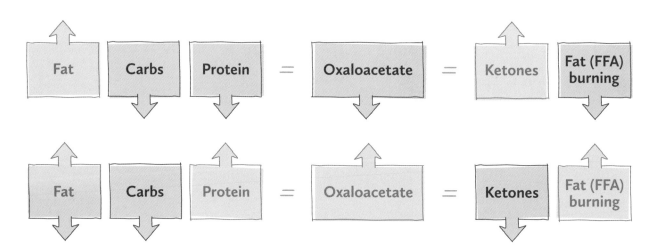

With oxaloacetate in short supply, the body must convert fat to ketones to be burned as fuel; it doesn't have a choice. Ketones are burned in the mitochondria without the use of oxaloacetate. This keeps the body's current supply of oxaloacetate burning all of the fat it can and running GNG. The body fuels everything else, primarily the brain, with ketones.

Since you need carbs or protein to make oxaloacetate, you can think of carbs and protein as the flames of a campfire. The logs represent fat (free fatty acids).

The logs (free fatty acids) are the fuel, and more fire (protein and/or carbs) means that more logs will burn!

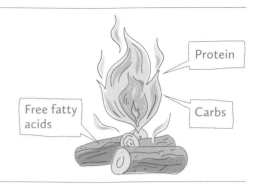

Protein

Carbs

Free fatty acids

Turning fat into ketones before burning those ketones as fuel is less efficient than burning fat for fuel directly. When you eat more protein, your ketone levels drop because the protein gives your body more precursors to make oxaloacetate. So now, fat goes through the Krebs cycle to be used for fuel instead of having to be turned into ketones first. Adding more protein to your diet allows your liver to work more efficiently and your body to burn fat for fuel more efficiently.

In this way, you can see that getting enough protein not only ensures that you won't lose muscle and can even build new muscle, but also provides your body with the oxaloacetate it needs to burn fat directly as fuel. The body no longer needs as many ketones to fuel itself. It just runs on the fat from your fat stores. In this state, your body is running much more efficiently.

Don't fear protein, and don't limit protein! You need protein to build and maintain muscle and to have enough substrates to make oxaloacetate so that you can burn more fat directly in your cells. Protein is the most essential macronutrient for health and weight loss, and the PSMF method makes sure you get enough of it.

Nutrient-Dense Foods

One of the great things about the PSMF method is that it focuses on some of the most nutrient-dense foods you can eat: animal proteins. This makes PSMF much different from any other type of fasting, like extended fasting, which is generally devoid of nutrients. Our bodies need vitamins and minerals along with complete proteins to thrive and to heal and reverse damage.

The following chart shows how a few plant "superfoods" stack up against beef and beef liver.

Nutrients in Plant "Superfoods" Compared to Animal Protein

Per Serving	Apples	Blueberries	Kale	Beef	Beef Liver
Calcium (mg)	9.1	4.5	63.4	11.0	11.0
Magnesium (mg)	7.3	4.5	15.0	19.0	18.0
Phosphorus (mg)	20.0	9.0	24.6	175.0	387.0
Potassium (mg)	163.8	57.8	200.6	370.0	380.0
Iron (mg)	0.2	0.2	0.8	3.3	8.8
Zinc (mg)	0.2	0.2	0.2	4.5	4.0
Selenium (mcg)	0.0	0.1	0.4	14.2	39.7
Vitamin A (IU)	69.2	40.5	13530.9	40.0	53400.0
Vitamin B6 (mg)	0.0	0.1	0.1	0.4	1.1
Vitamin B12 (mg)	0.0	0.0	0.0	2.0	11.0
Vitamin C (mg)	7.3	7.3	36.1	2.0	27.0
Vitamin D (IU)	0.0	0.0	0.0	7.0	19.0
Vitamin E (mg)	0.2	0.5	0.8	1.7	0.6
Niacin (mg)	0.2	0.3	0.4	4.8	17.0
Folate (mcg)	0.0	4.5	11.4	6.0	145.0

This next chart shows how various animal proteins complement one another, together making up a nutrient-rich profile. For example, beef has a decent amount of vitamin A, but not a lot. So, if you eat only beef, you won't get a great deal of vitamin A. However, if you add some eggs or a little beef liver to your beef, you'll end up with a huge amount of vitamin A plus some calcium. If you add pork, you'll get a boost of potassium and selenium. If you add chicken, you'll get quite a bit of magnesium. If you add salmon, you'll get a boost of vitamin D, vitamin E, and folate. You get the idea. By focusing on protein on PSMF days (and on keto days in general) and covering a range of animal proteins and eggs, you ensure a nutrient-dense and complete nutritional profile, supplying your body with the nutrients it needs to thrive and heal.

Nutrients in Animal Protein

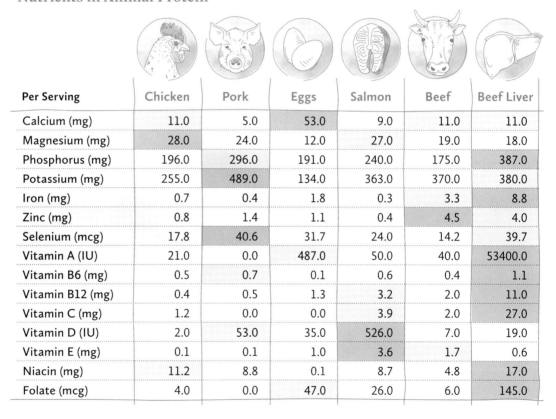

Per Serving	Chicken	Pork	Eggs	Salmon	Beef	Beef Liver
Calcium (mg)	11.0	5.0	53.0	9.0	11.0	11.0
Magnesium (mg)	28.0	24.0	12.0	27.0	19.0	18.0
Phosphorus (mg)	196.0	296.0	191.0	240.0	175.0	387.0
Potassium (mg)	255.0	489.0	134.0	363.0	370.0	380.0
Iron (mg)	0.7	0.4	1.8	0.3	3.3	8.8
Zinc (mg)	0.8	1.4	1.1	0.4	4.5	4.0
Selenium (mcg)	17.8	40.6	31.7	24.0	14.2	39.7
Vitamin A (IU)	21.0	0.0	487.0	50.0	40.0	53400.0
Vitamin B6 (mg)	0.5	0.7	0.1	0.6	0.4	1.1
Vitamin B12 (mg)	0.4	0.5	1.3	3.2	2.0	11.0
Vitamin C (mg)	1.2	0.0	0.0	3.9	2.0	27.0
Vitamin D (IU)	2.0	53.0	35.0	526.0	7.0	19.0
Vitamin E (mg)	0.1	0.1	1.0	3.6	1.7	0.6
Niacin (mg)	11.2	8.8	0.1	8.7	4.8	17.0
Folate (mcg)	4.0	0.0	47.0	26.0	6.0	145.0

This recommendation doesn't just apply to PSMF days. Focusing on animal proteins is an excellent strategy for anyone looking for nutrient-dense foods for health and healing. That is why we recommend emphasizing protein and hitting your protein goal each day for keto, too.

How much do you need to eat to get enough complete protein to build muscle? Let's compare broccoli (one of the highest sources of plant protein) to beef. To get to the threshold for starting muscle protein synthesis (mTOR), which is the body's process for turning amino acids into muscle, you need about 3.2 grams of leucine, an amino acid that signals mTOR to start building muscle from the protein you eat. You can get that amount by eating 7 ounces of steak or a whopping nine heads of broccoli!

How much is needed to trigger muscle building?

7 ounces	86 ounces (5.4 pounds)
1 sirloin steak	**9 heads of broccoli**

or

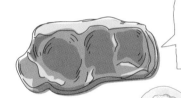

Also higher in 11 of 15 essential vitamins and minerals!

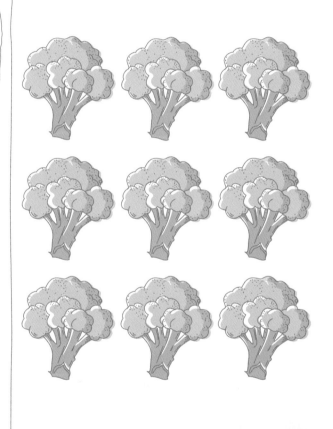

(per 100 g)	Broccoli	Beef
Calcium (mg)	47	11.0
Magnesium (mg)	18	19.0
Phosphorus (mg)	66	175.0
Potassium (mg)	316	370.0
Iron (mg)	0.7	3.3
Zinc (mg)	0.4	4.5
Selenium (mcg)	2.3	14.2
Vitamin A (IU)	623.0	40.0
Vitamin B6 (mg)	0.2	0.4
Vitamin B12 (mg)	0.0	2.0
Vitamin C (mg)	89.0	2.0
Vitamin D (IU)	0.0	7.0
Vitamin E (mg)	0.8	1.7
Niacin (mg)	0.6	4.8
Folate (mcg)	63.0	6.0

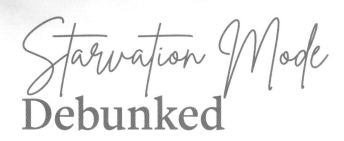

Starvation Mode Debunked

People often ask us about starvation mode and whether the PSMF method will create a situation—one they hear about and dread—where the body becomes resistant to weight loss after being starved for a long enough time.

The idea behind the so-called starvation mode is that if you restrict calories, your body "gets used to it" or "thinks this is the new normal" and then holds on to the calories it is getting, keeping you from losing fat even though you are eating in a caloric deficit. This is far from the truth.

We find it interesting that many of the people who believe in starvation mode also advocate doing three- or five-day fasts. If starvation mode were real, wouldn't the ultimate starvation (fasting, which brings in no calories at all) result in the body shutting down the metabolism completely and not burning any fat? Of course it wouldn't.

If this were true, the people who went through the 1845 famine in Ireland, where calorie intake for many was severely restricted for long periods, would not have become so skinny. In such conditions, wouldn't the body "hold on to calories" even more? In a 1992 study, researchers had one group eat 1,200 calories a day and the other 420 calories a day, only to find that the lower-calorie group lost 91 percent more weight.[14] Then there is the harshest starvation diet of them all, where a man fasted for 382 days in 1973.[15] Not only did he consistently lose weight throughout (about 0.33 kilograms per day), but his weight never really rebounded. We aren't suggesting that anyone starve themselves. In fact, the reason we recommend the PSMF method is that it gives you most of the benefits of fasting without the loss of lean mass. But these studies demonstrate that starvation mode is a myth. The idea that your body will hold on to stored fat even though you're eating in a caloric deficit just isn't accurate.

Another claim is that if you reduce your intake to, say, 1,200 or 1,100 calories a day, you will start to lose muscle. This will happen only if the calories you are eating are coming primarily from fat or carbs. If you get enough protein, you will not lose lean mass. This is another reason the PSMF method works so well.

[14]K. Arai et al., "Comparison of Clinical Usefulness of Very-Low-Calorie Diet and Supplemental Low-Calorie Diet," *American Journal of Clinical Nutrition* 56, no. 1 (1992): 275S–276S.

[15]W. K. Stewart and L. W. Fleming, "Features of a Successful Therapeutic Fast of 382 Days' Duration," *Postgraduate Medical Journal* 49, no. 569 (1973): 203–209.

We see it happen time and time again on our Facebook group: someone hits a stall even though their macros are on point and they're getting enough protein and limiting fat and carbs enough. The first comment people make to them is, "You need to eat more." The idea that you can lose more weight by eating more food every day has never made sense to us. How well did that work over the last 20 years that made you put on the extra weight to begin with?

That being said, we understand that when people limit their calories for a certain period of time, they really do experience a shift in how their bodies burn calories, and they have to eat fewer calories to maintain or lose weight. However, what they're experiencing isn't starvation mode. Instead, there are some factors at play, and they are as follows.

Miscalculation of Caloric Intake

Some people say, "But starvation mode is real—it happened to me! I can only eat 1,500 calories now, or I gain weight." It's worth noting that, on average, people underestimate the calories they consume by about 40 percent.[16] This means they eat far more than they think they do because they do not accurately weigh and track their food. If you weigh your food and count every gram, what you thought was 1,500 calories is probably more like 2,500 calories.

This is quite common and feeds into the myth of starvation mode. We see people posting on social media, "Here is my day; I ate about 1,500 calories." But on closer examination, you see four meals plus a dessert that total at least 2,500 calories. For a typical woman who isn't very active, 2,500 calories a day would result in a weight gain in most cases.

When you focus on protein, you eat nutrient-dense foods like meat. It can look like a lot less food than the processed foods in a standard American diet, but you get so many vitamins and minerals from animal proteins.

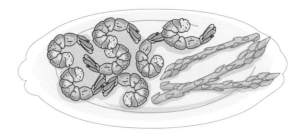

---

[16]S. W. Lichtman et al., "Discrepancy between Self-Reported and Actual Caloric Intake and Exercise in Obese Subjects," *New England Journal of Medicine* 31, no. 27 (1992): 1893–1898.

Metabolic Adaptation

Metabolic adaptation is where the body reduces its metabolic thermogenesis based on the reduction of calories in the diet for an extended period. Your basal metabolic rate, or BMR, is the number of calories your body needs each day to live in a state of rest, to fuel cells and do autophagy, as well as to build and repair muscle and other tissues and do all of the things that keep you alive (heart beating, breathing, etc.). This means that if you eat in a large calorie deficit for months at a time, your BMR will drop, and you will require fewer calories to maintain or even fewer calories to lose weight.

This is where overfeeding days can be a good idea. Getting 400 to 600 extra calories from fat and protein can help limit metabolic adaption. We have always promoted implementing an overfeeding day occasionally to help reduce metabolic adaptation. We recommend you do this based on your body's needs, adding overfeeding days occasionally when you are extra hungry. Doing this every other week, or even every week, can be helpful for some people, whereas others may need to keep it to one day a month or so. In general, just go by what your body tells you. If you experience extra hunger one day, add some protein and fat. But don't do it every day, as that would limit your weight-loss results.

You may be thinking, "What's the difference between metabolic adaptation and starvation mode, then?" The idea behind starvation mode is that if you drop your caloric intake to a certain level—1,200 a day or whatever—your body will freak out and refuse to lose weight, or even start gaining weight. However, when we look at this through the lens of metabolic adaptation, what's really happening when you lose weight is that your calorie expenditure will slow down some, and thus you need to eat less to maintain. But it isn't due to "starvation mode."

Just think about losing 100 pounds. Now, we're talking about 100 pounds you no longer need to carry around all day; we're talking about many fat cells that don't need energy all day. It's like going from exercising while wearing a 100-pound backpack to exercising without it. The difference in energy required to perform even basic tasks is enormous! This means you will naturally require fewer calories to maintain your new weight.

Also, restricting calories a lot, like under 1,000 calories a day, for months and months, can result in incremental reductions or adaptions to the metabolism. But overfeeding days will help reduce those effects. Adding overfeeding days limits metabolic adaptation and keeps the metabolism going. That being said, if weight loss is your goal, you should never eat if you're not hungry. Overfeeding based on your hunger signals instead of planning them on specific days is a better strategy. However, if you simply never get hungry, add an occasional overfeeding day to prevent too much adaption.

Metabolic adaptation will happen with weight loss, regardless of which diet you use to lose the weight: low carb, low fat, or anything else. Therefore, the choice is to stay obese and suffer the consequences or to lose weight and, as a result of not having to carry around all that extra weight, eat slightly fewer calories in maintenance. What we're emphasizing here is the need to see eating keto, carnivore, or low carb as a lifestyle, not a diet. That is how you succeed long term. Thinking you can lose the weight with keto and then go back to the old habits that made you gain the weight in the first place, without gaining it all back again, is just not realistic. Instead, you must stick with this lifestyle and find ways to enjoy the foods you love while keeping yourself on track.

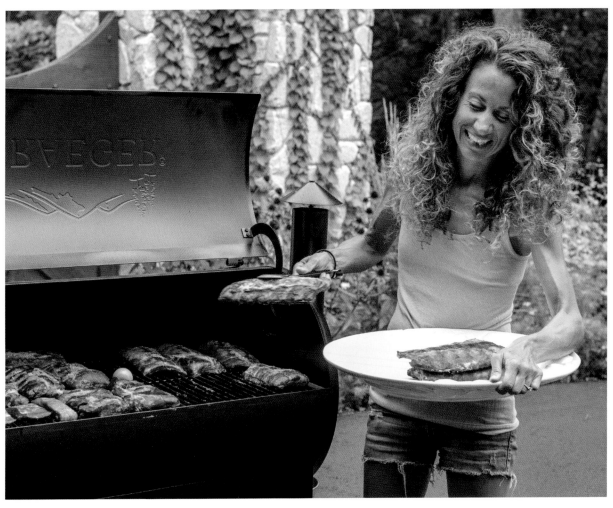

Doing the PSMF Method the Wrong Way

Protein-sparing modified fasting is a tool, and it can be used incorrectly. PSMF days are very low in calories, so doing them too often, or when you don't have a lot of body fat to lose, can lead to negative consequences.

For example, if you are a lean person who is only 5 or 10 pounds from your goal weight, you want to limit PSMF days to perhaps one a week. This is because your body needs fuel, and if you lower dietary energy when you don't have much on your body, your body will start converting protein to fuel, which means you will lose muscle.

Also, if your goal is to control seizures or Alzheimer's, where higher blood ketones are a good thing, the PSMF method may not be for you. You might need to eat more fat to make enough ketones to keep your symptoms at bay.

If you have a lot of weight to lose, like 50 pounds or more, adding one to three days a week of PSMF is a good idea. But we do not recommend doing it every day or even five days a week for extended periods. While the PSMF method uses nutrient-dense foods, you just aren't eating a lot, so the more days a week you follow the PSMF method, the harder it is to get the vitamins and minerals that your body needs. Mixing it up and doing PSMF a couple of days a week is a better plan.

If you are doing three PSMF days a week, adding one overfeeding day once a week or every other week is a good idea. That will give you the results you're looking for while limiting metabolic adaptation and preserving your lean mass.

I did extended fasting (for 72 hours, or two 42-hour fasts a week) for a while, and I almost always gained back 90 percent of what I "lost." In addition, I had massive hair loss, clear nails, and a bad stomach whenever I broke my fast. Switching to PSMF, I get slightly less dramatic weight-loss results overall but more significant measurement changes (so I'm assuming fat loss without muscle loss), all without any of the negative side effects.

I am glad that fasting helped break my hangry issues and let me know that I can survive without food if I have to. But if I am going to choose what is healthiest for myself—and I do have a choice—I will stick to PSMF from now on when fasting is needed to reach my goals.

— Rachel

Implementing the PSMF Method

Protein-sparing modified fasting isn't something you want to do every day; you want to do it a couple of days a week—occasionally as needed—to speed up fat loss or to break a stall. Although you are eating some of the most nutrient-dense foods, you are eating very little—typically about 600 to 700 calories—so you aren't getting many vitamins and minerals that your body needs. So try implementing only one or two PSMF days a week and then use your regular fat-loss keto or carnivore macros the other days (like in Maria's book *The 30-Day Ketogenic Cleanse,* which is dairy-free and nut-free to help with healing). You can get keto, carnivore, and PSMF macros with our free calculator on our blog, KetoMaria.com.

If you want to be aggressive, you could do up to four days a week of PSMF for a while. But PSMF is a tool to use when you want to speed up weight loss or break a stall, not all the time.

Calculate Your Target Macros

The PSMF method is more structured than several other types of fasting, and for it to be as effective as possible, precision is required. That said, PSMF days are very similar for everyone; it's the protein intake that can vary from one person to another.

In general, you want to have about 10 grams or fewer of total carbs—or even none at all—and 20 to 30 grams or so of fat, the bare minimum to help your body absorb fat-soluble vitamins and to make healthy hormones.

Protein, on the other hand, depends on you and your lean mass. The taller you are or the more muscle you have, the more protein you need. For a typical adult (under the age of 60 or so), we typically recommend about 0.8 times your lean mass for your protein goal in grams. This gives you enough protein to maintain and build lean mass. If you are younger, or if you are older than 60, you need even more protein. Kids need extra protein to fuel growth; for example, toddlers need about 2.0 times their lean mass in grams of protein a day. Newborn babies get about 2.6 times their lean mass in grams of protein a day when breastfed!

As we age, our bodies require even more protein to maintain lean mass. So if you're over 60, you will want 1.0 to 1.2 times your lean mass; if over 70, 1.2 to 1.4 times your lean mass. We have factored all this into our keto calculator at https://mariamindbodyhealth.com/calculator/.

On PSMF, we recommend that a typical adult under 60 years of age increase their protein amount to about 1.0 times lean mass. Hitting your normal goal (0.8 times lean mass) is fine if you are not hungry. However, if hunger is an issue, a higher protein amount is advised.

Let's look at an example for a typical woman under 60 years of age who is 5 feet, 4 inches tall, weighs 170 pounds, and has 38 percent body fat. This means she has 105 pounds of lean mass.

$$170 \times 0.38 = 64.6 \text{ pounds of body fat}$$

$$170 - 64.6 = 105.4 \text{ pounds of lean mass}$$

$$105 \times 1.0 = 105 \text{ grams of protein}$$

Her macros for her PSMF days would be little to no carbs, 105 grams of protein, and about 30 grams of fat. What does that look like in the body when we account for the thermic effect of food? Here we've assumed 0 grams of carbs for simplification:

$$30 \text{ grams of fat} = 270 \text{ calories } (\textit{1 gram of fat is 9 calories})$$

$$270 - \text{TEF of 3 percent} = 262 \text{ effective calories}$$

$$105 \text{ grams of protein} = 420 \text{ calories } (\textit{1 gram of protein is 4 calories})$$

$$420 - \text{TEF of 25 percent} = 315 \text{ effective calories}$$

As you can see, this is like fasting while preserving lean mass because she is getting only about 690 total calories, and only about 577 (262 + 315) of those calories are useful because of the thermic effect of food. So she will get enough protein to preserve lean body mass, but she will have to use a lot of stored fat to fuel her body. This is what makes the PSMF method such an excellent tool for accelerating weight loss or breaking a stall. And because of the satiating properties of protein and stable blood glucose, she will not be hungry or have severe cravings like she would if she ate only this many calories of carbohydrate.

Being keto-adapted before doing PSMF is helpful, though not required; it makes it much easier to do PSMF days without hunger issues. When you are fully keto-adapted (after four to six weeks or so on strict keto), your body will be very efficient at tapping into its stored body fat for fuel.

Take Advantage of the Protein/Energy Ratio

The protein to energy ratio (P/E) is a helpful measure for picking the right foods for PSMF days. P/E is simply the grams of protein in a food divided by the grams of energy in that food. This gives you the ratio of how much protein there is in a food compared to how much energy there is (carbs and fat). The higher a food's P/E value, the better it is for fat loss.

In general, a P/E above 1.0 is good for weight loss—above 2.0 is even better. Anything above 3.0 is getting into a range that is great for PSMF days. You could combine a meal that is 2.0 with another meal that is 6.0 and still have a great fast if the resulting macros fit the guidelines for PSMF days.

Here is an example. A 4-ounce boneless, skinless chicken breast contains about 25 grams of protein, 4 grams of fat, and 0 grams of carbohydrate. The resulting P/E would be

$$P/E = (25)/(4+0) = 6.25$$

As you can see, the P/E of chicken breast is 6.25, which is very good for PSMF days.

While P/E is a great tool to help you determine whether a food will be good for fat loss, you still need to consider where the energy comes from. Energy from fat is much better than energy from sugar. If a food has a high P/E ratio but is also high in sugar, it will drive glucose up and result in more hunger and cravings.

Also, be careful about subtracting fiber from the P/E ratio, which is how it is typically done by Dr. Ted Naiman, who wrote the book *The P:E Diet.* This practice might be fine for whole foods like mushrooms, but it can get you into trouble with processed foods. Many product labels these days use the fiber numbers to hide things such as soluble corn fiber, which spikes blood sugar almost as much as sugar does. So when you calculate the P/E of a processed food, go with the total carbs instead of net carbs. However, since this book is all whole foods–based, we used the traditional calculation for the P/E ratio.

Focus on High-Quality Proteins for PSMF Days

The PSMF method focuses on animal proteins, as they are the foods highest in complete proteins. However, plant foods that are low in carbs and fat, such as asparagus, broccoli, cabbage, cauliflower, eggplant, garlic, lettuce, mushrooms, tomatoes, and spices, can be added to meals as long as the macros remain in line.

Because animal proteins have very little to no carbohydrate, you just have to look at the fat content to determine if they are good for PSMF days. Certain cuts of meat are better than others for PSMF. In general, the lower the fat and the higher the P/E, the better a cut is.

Here is a list of the best cuts for PSMF sorted by P/E ratio.

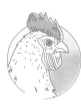

Poultry (4 ounces)	Calories	Fat	Protein	Carbs	P/E Ratio
Chicken gizzards	175	3.0	34.5	0	11.50
Chicken breast, skinless	138	4.0	25.0	0	6.25
Chicken giblets (kidney)	178	5.1	30.8	0	6.04
Chicken liver	189	7.4	27.7	1.0	3.74
Chicken breast, skin-on	200	8.4	31.0	0	3.69
Chicken heart	210	9.0	30.0	0.1	3.33
Chicken leg, skinless	210	9.5	30.7	0	3.23
Pheasant	200	10.5	25.7	0	2.45
Chicken drums	178	9.9	22.0	0	2.22
Turkey	175	9.9	21.0	0	2.12
Chicken leg, skin-on	255	15.2	29.4	0	1.93
Chicken thigh, skinless	165	10.0	19.0	0	1.90
Duck	228	13.9	26.3	0	1.89
Chicken thigh, skin-on	275	17.6	28.3	0	1.61
Chicken wings	320	22.0	30.4	0	1.38
Chicken feet	244	16.6	22.0	0.2	1.33
Game hen	220	16.0	19.0	0	1.19
Goose	340	24.9	28.5	0	1.14
Chicken skin	514	46.0	23.0	0	0.50

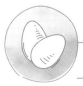

Eggs	Calories	Fat	Protein	Carbs	P/E Ratio
Egg white (1 large)	17.4	0.06	3.64	0.24	12.13
Egg (1 large)*	68.2	4.7	5.5	0.5	1.07

*Be careful; yolks add fat and lower P/E quickly!

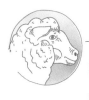

Goat & Lamb (4 ounces)	Calories	Fat	Protein	Carbs	P/E Ratio
Goat ribs	162	3.4	30.7	0	9.03
Goat meat	162	3.4	30.7	0	9.03
Lamb oysters (testicles)	154	3.4	29.7	1.14	6.54
Goat oysters (testicles)	154	3.4	29.7	1.14	6.54
Goat liver	217	5.9	33.0	5.8	2.82
Lamb liver	250	10.0	34.7	2.87	2.70
Lamb, ground	313	22.7	25.5	0	1.12
Lamb chops	313	22.7	25.5	0	1.12

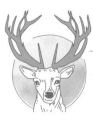

Wild Game (4 ounces)	Calories	Fat	Protein	Carbs	P/E Ratio
Venison loin*	169	2.7	34.3	0	12.85
Elk steak	168	3.2	34.7	0	10.84
Venison steak	179	3.6	34.3	0	9.53
Venison roast	179	3.6	34.3	0	9.53
Bison top round steak	138	2.8	26.4	0	9.43
Rabbit meat	196	4.0	37.4	0	9.35
Elk loin	189	4.4	35.0	0	7.95
Bison chuck shoulder	219	6.0	38.3	0	6.38
Venison heart	187	5.4	32.3	0	5.80
Bison rib-eye	200	6.4	33.4	0	5.22
Bison top sirloin	194	6.4	31.8	0	4.97
Venison liver	196	8.0	28.0	0	3.50
Venison, ground	212	9.3	30.0	0	3.23
Elk, ground	219	9.9	30.2	0	3.05
Bison, ground	166	8.2	23.0	0	2.80
Bison liver	241	5.3	33.3	6.7	2.78
Bear meat	186	9.4	22.8	0	2.43
Bison heart	239	16.0	22.7	0	1.42

*Venison refers specifically to deer in this case.

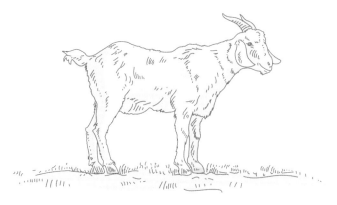

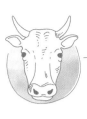

Beef (4 ounces)	Calories	Fat	Protein	Carbs	P/E Ratio
Tenderloin steak	115	3.0	22.2	0	7.40
Testicles	154	3.4	29.7	1.14	6.54
Heart	187	5.4	32.2	0.2	5.96
Kidney	179	5.3	31.0	0	5.85
Shank cross cut	215	6.7	38.7	0	5.80
Sirloin tip side steak	190	6.0	34.0	0	5.67
Liver	216	6.0	33.0	5.8	5.50
Sirloin tip center steak	190	7.0	31.0	0	4.43
Sirloin tip center roast	190	7.0	31.0	0	4.43
Shoulder pot roast	185	7.0	30.7	0	4.38
Flank steak	200	8.0	32.0	0	4.00
Round tip steak	150	6.0	23.5	0	3.92
Shoulder petite tender medallions	150	7.0	22.0	0	3.14
Shoulder petite tender	150	7.0	22.0	0	3.14
Tenderloin roast	180	8.0	25.0	0	3.13
Shoulder center ranch steak	152	8.0	24.0	0	3.00
Tripe (intestines)	107	4.6	13.3	2.3	2.89
Eye of round steak	182	9.0	25.0	0	2.78
Top round steak	180	9.0	25.0	0	2.78
Chuck steak, boneless	160	8.0	22.0	0	2.75
Eye of round roast	253	13.4	32.0	0	2.39
Tri-tip steak	200	11.0	23.0	0	2.09
Chuck pot roast, boneless	240	14.0	28.0	0	2.00
Chuck pot roast, 7-bone	240	14.0	28.0	0	2.00
Shoulder steak	204	12.0	24.0	0	2.00
Brisket, flat cut	245	14.7	28.0	0	1.91
Round tip roast	199	12.0	22.9	0	1.91
Shoulder top blade steak	204	13.0	22.0	0	1.69
Shoulder top blade flat iron steak	204	13.0	22.0	0	1.69
Bottom round roast	220	14.0	23.0	0	1.64
Bottom round steak	220	14.0	23.0	0	1.64
Skirt steak	255	16.5	27.0	0	1.64
Top sirloin steak	240	16.0	22.0	0	1.38
T-bone	170	12.2	15.8	0	1.30
Chuck eye steak	250	18.0	21.0	0	1.17
Brains	171	11.9	13.2	1.7	1.11
Top loin steak, bone-in	270	20.0	21.0	0	1.05
Top loin steak, boneless	270	20.0	21.0	0	1.05
Rib roast	373	28.0	27.0	0	0.96
Porterhouse	280	22.0	21.0	0	0.95
Sweetbreads	362	28.3	25.0	0	0.88
Tongue	322	25.3	22.0	0	0.87
Rib-eye steak	310	25.0	20.0	0	0.80
Back ribs	310	26.0	19.0	0	0.73
Tri-tip roast	340	29.0	18.0	0	0.62
Short ribs, boneless	440	41.0	16.0	0	0.39

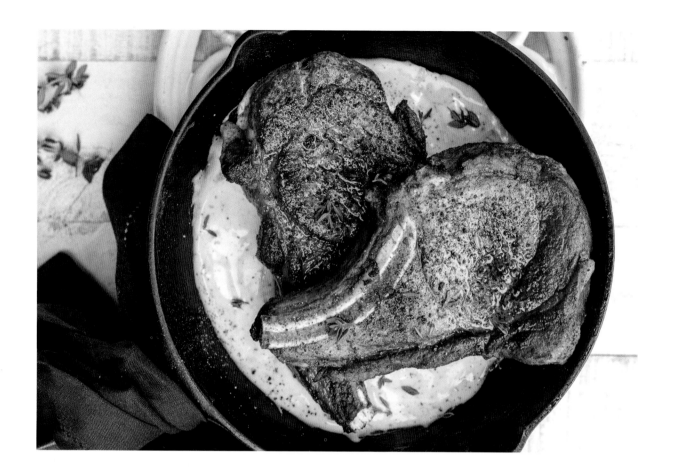

Pork (4 ounces)	Calories	Fat	Protein	Carbs	P/E Ratio
Tenderloin	158	4.0	30.0	0	7.50
Liver	187	5.0	29.5	4.3	5.90
Kidney	171	5.3	28.8	0	5.43
Heart	168	5.7	26.8	0.5	4.70
Chop	241	12.0	33.0	0	2.75
Rump	280	16.2	32.8	0	2.02
Loin	265	15.5	30.8	0	1.99
Middle ribs (country style)	245	16.0	25.0	0	1.56
Leg ham	305	20.0	30.4	0	1.52
Ears	188	12.3	18.0	0.2	1.46
Tongue	307	21.0	27.3	0	1.30
Brains	156	11.0	14.0	0	1.27
Butt	240	18.0	19.0	0	1.06
Cracklings (pork rinds)	530	40.0	39.0	1.9	0.98
Bacon	600	47.2	41.8	0	0.89
Shoulder	285	23.0	19.0	0	0.83
Hocks	285	24.0	17.0	0	0.71
Loin back ribs (baby back ribs)	315	27.0	18.0	0	0.67
Belly	588	60.0	10.4	0	0.17

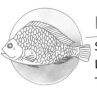

Fish & Seafood (4 ounces)	Calories	Fat	Protein	Carbs	P/E Ratio
Shrimp	112	0.32	27.2	0.23	49.45
Langostino	93	0.67	21.3	0	31.79
Tuna (canned)	149	1.06	32.91	0	31.05
Northern pike	128	1.0	28	0	28.00
Cod	113	1.0	26	0	26.00
Orange roughy	119	1.0	25.7	0	25.70
Crab	94	0.84	20.28	0	24.14
Tuna (yellowfin)	150	1.5	34	0	22.67
Lobster	101	1.0	22	0	22.67
Perch	132	1.34	28.2	0	22.00
Bluegill	133	1.34	28.2	0	21.04
Crappie	132	1.34	28.2	0	21.04
Mahi mahi	100	1.0	21.0	0	21.00
Grouper	134	1.5	28.2	0	18.80
Crayfish (crawfish)	93	1.4	19.0	0	13.57
Barramundi	110	2.0	23.0	0	11.50
Tilapia	145	3.0	29.7	0	9.90
Monkfish	110	2.2	21.1	0	9.59
Sea bass	135	3.0	27.0	0	9.00
Halibut	155	3.5	30.7	0	8.77
Salmon roe (ikura)	185	4.0	34.3	0	8.58
Catfish	119	3.2	20.9	0	6.53
Flounder	97.5	2.7	17.3	0	6.41
Turbot	138	4.3	23.3	0	5.42
Octopus	186	2.4	33.8	5.0	4.57
Squid	119	1.8	20.3	4.0	3.50
Salmon	206	9.0	31.0	0	3.44
Scallops	126	1.0	23.0	6.0	3.29
Trout	190	8.6	28.0	0	3.26
Swordfish	195	9.0	26.6	0	2.96
Walleye	156	7.5	22.0	0	2.93
Arctic char	208	10.0	29.0	0	2.90
Cockle	90	0.8	15.3	5.3	2.50
Fish livers	118	5.0	12.5	5.8	2.50
Sardines	139	7.5	18.0	0.0	2.40
Clams	161	6.7	27.5	6.7	2.05
Mussels	195	5.0	27.0	8.38	2.02
Sea urchin	137	5.6	18.3	3.9	1.93
Anchovies	256	15.9	28.0	0	1.76
Eel	267	17.0	26.8	0	1.58
Mackerel	290	20.3	27.0	0	1.33
Oysters	92	2.6	10.7	5.6	1.30
Herring	283.5	20.2	23.8	0.0	1.18
Caviar	299	20.3	27.9	4.54	1.12
Escargot	21.6	0.2	1.3	3.5	0.35

Make the Most of Your PSMF Days

As we have emphasized throughout this introduction, the PSMF method is a wonderful tool for speeding up weight loss and healing. While getting your macros right contributes to about 90 percent of your weight-loss success, a few things can help tip the scales to ensure the best results. Here are some important tips that will help you make the most of your PSMF days:

 Avoid too much strenuous exercise. Exercise is great, but too much intense exercise can increase blood sugar, which results in a glucose drop to compensate. Falling glucose increases hunger. Stick to leisurely walks or gentle yoga.

 Cut out all caffeinated drinks. Caffeine increases blood sugar by 8 percent, and later in the day, when blood sugar starts to fall, it will cause hunger and sugar cravings. Caffeine also lowers insulin sensitivity. In fact, if you cut out coffee, you likely will be able to lose weight if you have been stuck for a while—not to mention enjoy better-quality sleep (see the next tip)!

 Get adequate sleep. Sleep is essential to weight loss and health. We used to ask our clients, "Do you sleep well?" However, we had to change the question to, "How long do you sleep?" Clients often responded to our question about sleeping well with a "yes," but when we asked how long they slept, they often said five or six hours. You need at least eight hours of good sleep to repair your body and thrive. Sleep deprivation increases sugar cravings and can make weight loss very difficult.

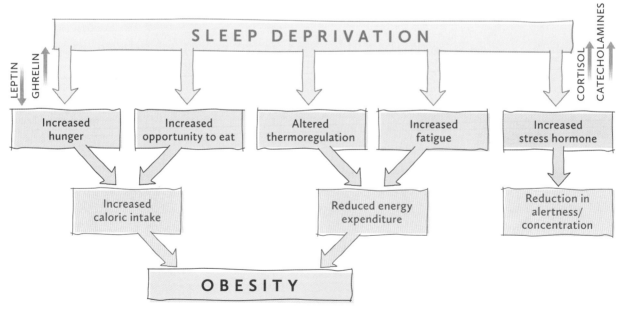

Getting good sleep is one of the most important things you can do for long-term health and weight loss. When you don't get good sleep, your hunger hormones will cause you to crave and eat more food the next day. Here are some tips for getting a good night's sleep:

Eliminate sugar to stabilize your blood sugar and avoid a drop in the middle of the night, which will wake you up.

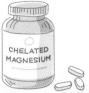

Take chelated magnesium, such as glycinate or topical magnesium, about an hour before bed. Magnesium is very calming and often helps with sleep.

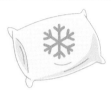

Make your bedroom cooler. A cooler environment helps with sleep.

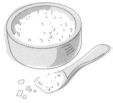

Use an Epsom salt bath or a cool foot soak. It's another way to get magnesium. (Avoid hot foot soaks; cool soaks help make the mitochondria more efficient in oxidizing fat.)

Try essential oils, such as lavender oil—a dab of it on the big toe can help with sleep.

Add salt before bed, as low salt will cause poor sleep. This is especially helpful if you get up to urinate often during the night. Take a sodium capsule or an electrolyte shot before bed.

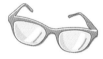

Wear blue-blocking glasses at night to block out blue light from your TV, computer, and smartphone. Blocking blue light in the evening allows the body to produce its sleep hormone, melatonin, naturally.

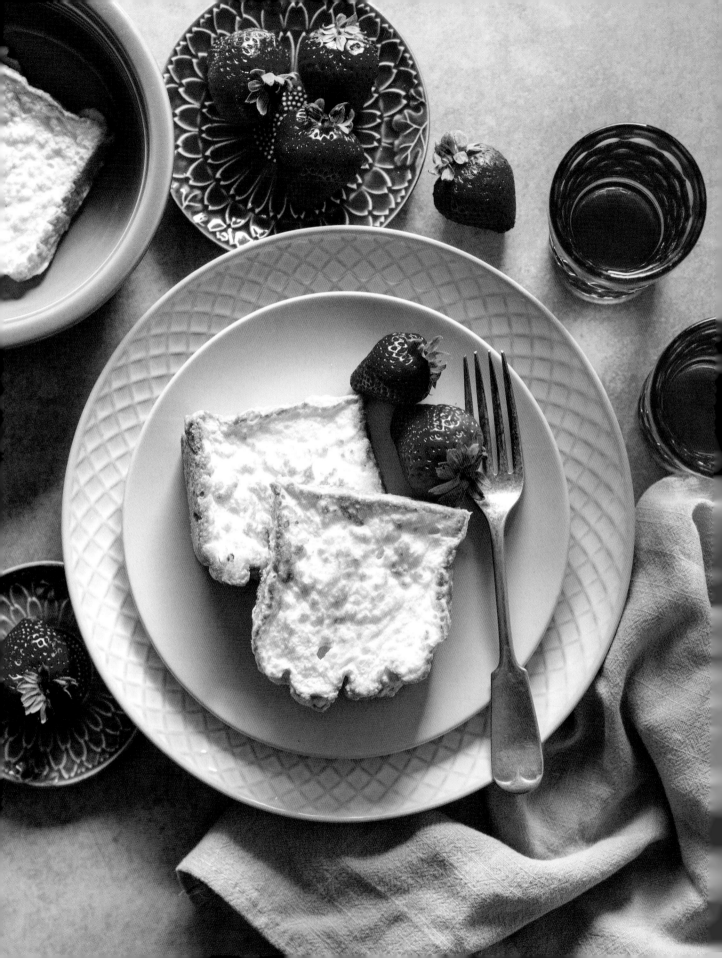

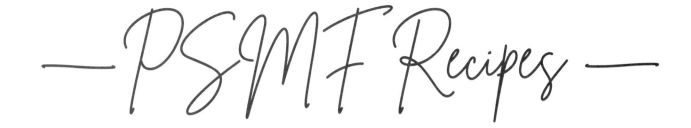

PSMF Recipes

The protein-sparing modified fast is traditionally seen as boring—eating nothing but chicken breasts or something like that. This is far from the truth! Maria is the ultimate recipe wizard, and in this book, you will see that PSMF can be flavorful, inviting, and even comforting.

These recipes provide truly innovative methods for transforming basic ingredients, like eggs, into pudding, bread, and even ice cream. PSMF is anything but boring when done the Emmerich way!

Note: You'll find these icons in the recipes as applicable:

 Dairy free

 Egg free

 Nut free

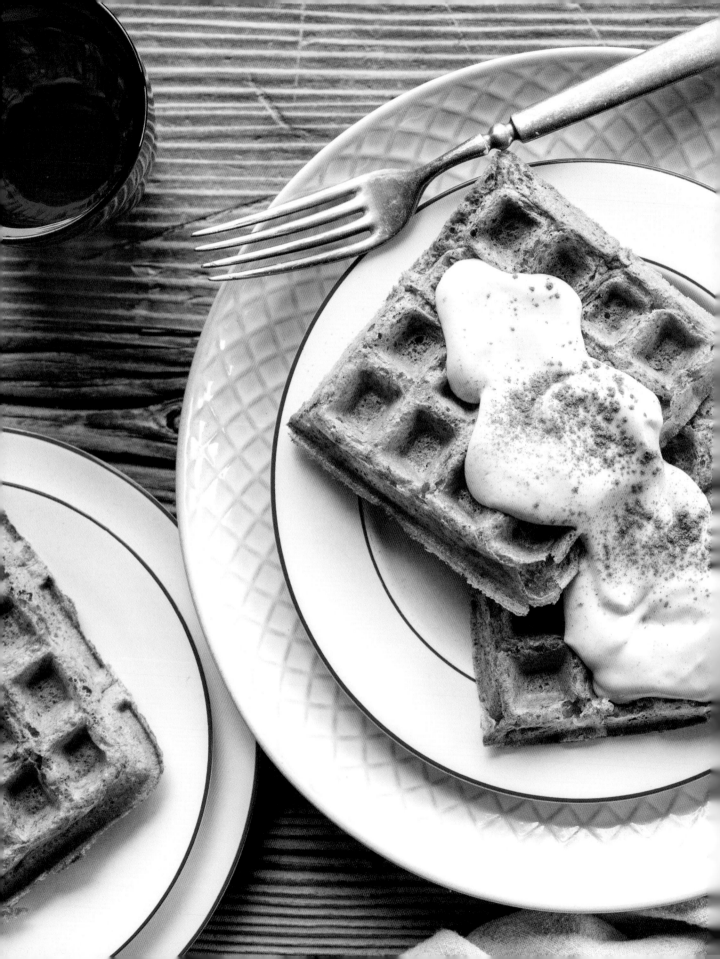

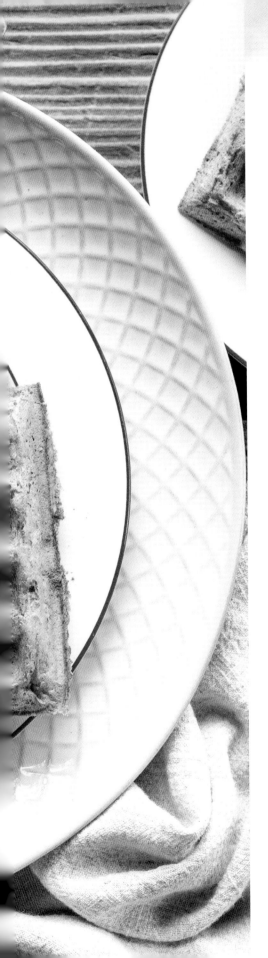

chapter 1
Breakfast

Turkey Frittata / 54

Ham Omelet / 56

Soufflé Omelet with Ham and Chives / 58

Steak and Eggs / 60

Breakfast Patties / 62

Breakfast Sammie / 64

Protein-Sparing Pancakes / 66

Savory Dutch Baby with Lox / 68

Apple Dutch Baby / 70

Cinnamon Roll Waffles / 72

Classic French Toast / 74

Strawberry Angel Food French Toast / 76

Minute Breakfast Muffins / 78

French Toast Porridge / 80

Chocolate Hot Breakfast Cereal / 82

Chocolate Breakfast Pudding / 84

Strawberry Shake / 86

Orange Creamsicle Smoothie / 88

Turkey Frittata

  yield: 2 servings • prep time: 5 minutes • cook time: 20 minutes

Although the flavors of turkey, thyme, and sage remind us of Thanksgiving, this comforting breakfast can be enjoyed at any time of the year or day.

Duck fat spray or coconut oil spray, for greasing

1 cup diced cooked boneless, skinless turkey breast

8 large egg whites, lightly beaten

½ teaspoon dried thyme leaves

½ teaspoon dried rubbed sage

½ teaspoon onion salt or fine sea salt

¼ teaspoon freshly ground black pepper

1. Preheat the oven to 350°F. Lightly grease a 6-inch cake pan with duck fat spray.

2. Put all of the ingredients in a medium-sized bowl and stir to combine, then pour the mixture into the prepared pan. Bake until set in the center, 20 to 24 minutes. Cut into wedges and serve warm.

3. Leftovers can be stored in an airtight container in the refrigerator for up to 4 days. To reheat, place in a 350°F oven for a few minutes, until warmed through.

P/E ratio **3.5** • calories **206** • fat **4g** • protein **39g** • carbs **1g** • fiber **0.3g**

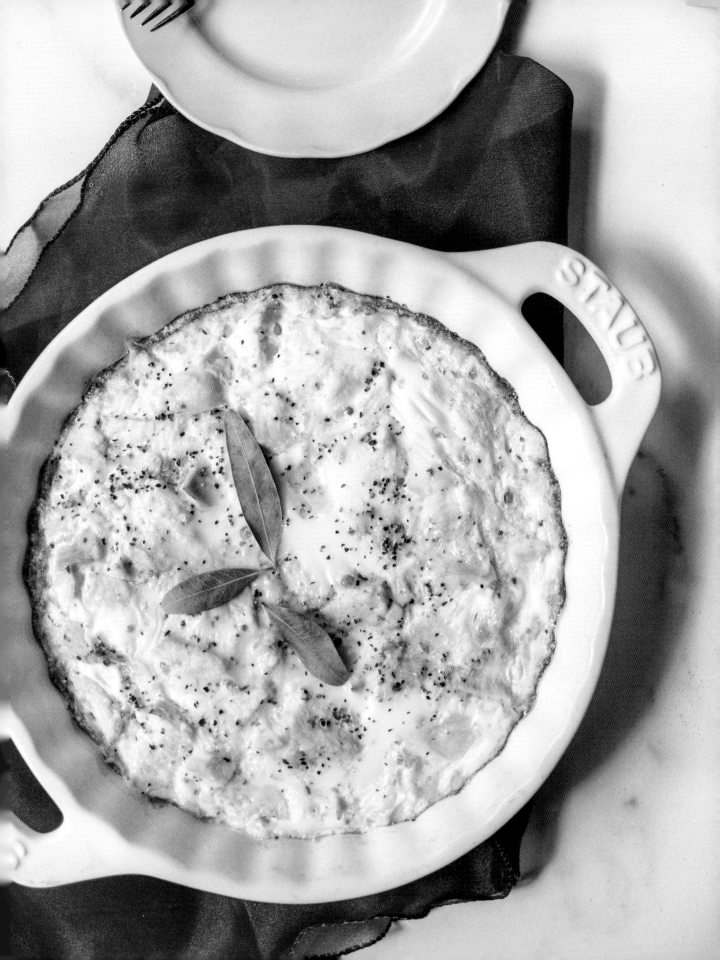

Ham
Omelet

  yield: 1 serving • prep time: 5 minutes • cook time: 5 minutes

4 large egg whites

1 tablespoon water

⅛ teaspoon fine sea salt

⅛ teaspoon freshly ground black pepper

1 teaspoon coconut oil (preferably butter-flavored)

2 ounces 95% lean ham, chopped

Chopped fresh chives, for garnish (optional)

Protein-Sparing Bread (page 270), for serving (optional)

1. Put the egg whites, water, salt, and pepper in a small bowl and beat with a fork until combined.

2. Melt the oil in a small nonstick skillet over medium-low heat. Pour in the egg white mixture and gently stir with a rubber spatula for a few seconds as if you were making scrambled eggs. Tilt the pan so the egg mixture covers the entire cooking surface. Adjust the heat as needed to prevent browning or burning. Continue cooking until the eggs are set on the bottom but still slightly liquid on top, about 1 minute more.

3. Remove the skillet from the heat. Spread the ham across the center of the omelet. Gently lift one side of the omelet with the spatula to fold it in half and press down lightly. Garnish with chives, if using. Serve warm with Protein-Sparing Bread, if desired.

P/E ratio **1.8** • calories **245** • fat **14g** • protein **27g** • carbs **1g** • fiber **0.1g**

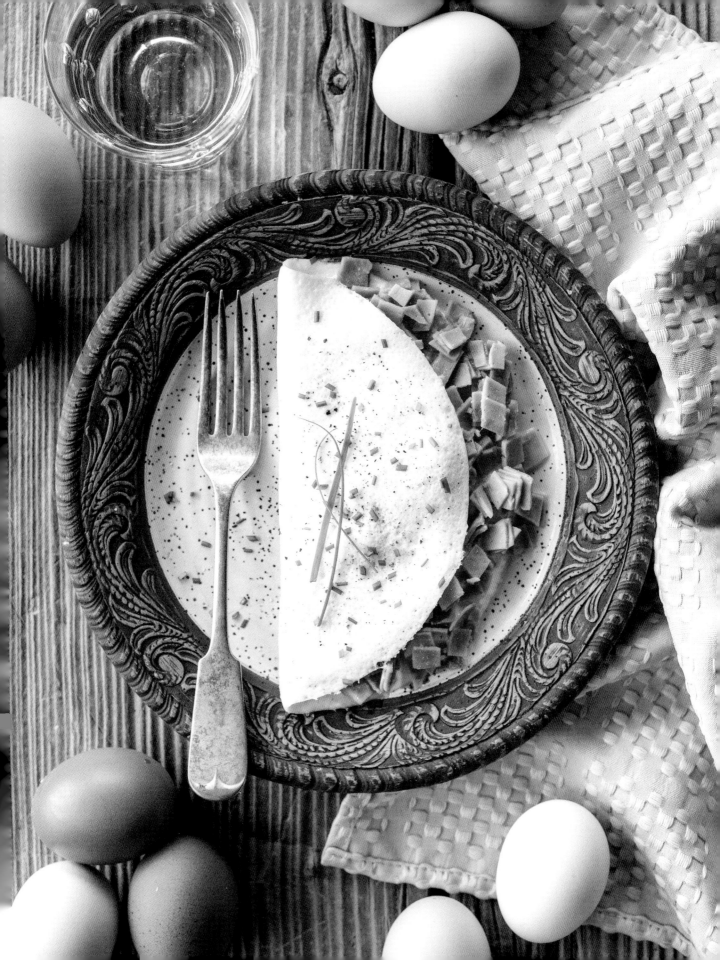

Soufflé Omelet
with Ham and Chives

  yield: 1 serving • prep time: 5 minutes • cook time: 7 minutes

Duck fat spray or coconut oil spray, for greasing

5 large egg whites

1 large egg yolk, lightly beaten

¼ cup diced 95% lean ham

2 tablespoons chopped fresh chives

½ teaspoon fine sea salt

1. Preheat the oven to 375°F. Lightly grease a 7-inch pie dish with duck fat spray.

2. Place the egg whites in a medium-sized bowl and beat with an electric hand mixer on high speed until stiff peaks form. Gently fold in the yolk, ham, chives, and salt, being careful not to deflate the whites.

3. Pour the egg mixture into the prepared pie dish. Bake until set but still slightly soft in the center, 7 to 9 minutes. Serve immediately.

P/E ratio **2.2** • calories **227** • fat **11g** • protein **28g** • carbs **2g** • fiber **0.2g**

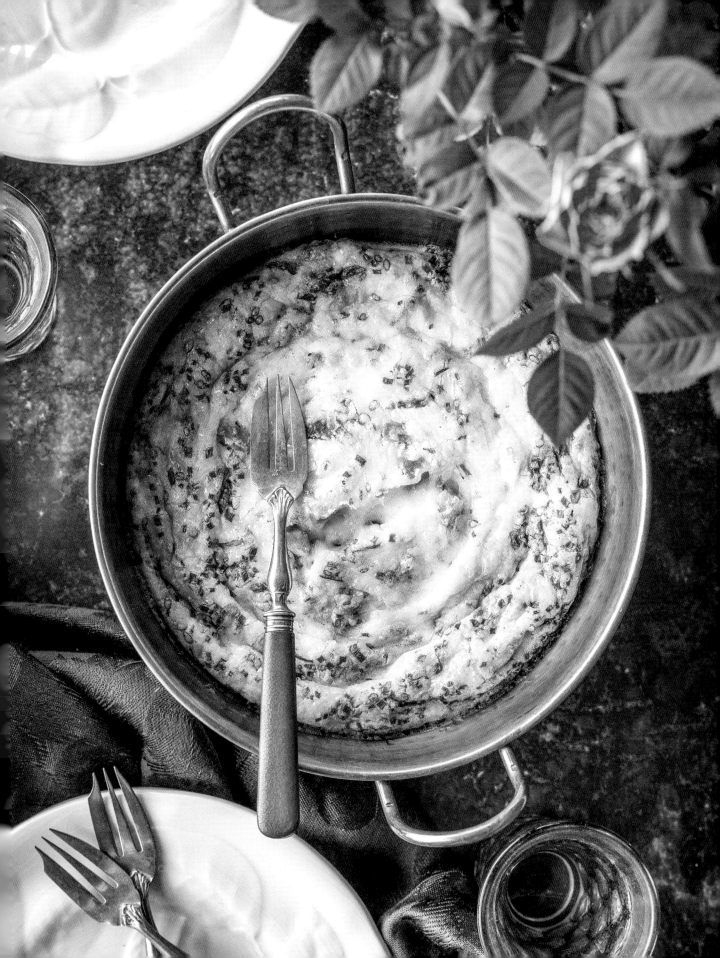

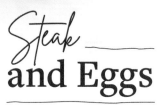

Steak and Eggs

  yield: 2 servings • prep time: 5 minutes, plus 10 minutes to rest • cook time: 10 minutes

You can never go wrong with the classic breakfast combo of steak and eggs. For PSMF days, stick with egg whites, but on regular eating days, feel free to cook a whole egg. Add a couple of strips of bacon if you are extra hungry!

2 (4-ounce) venison or beef tenderloin steaks

Fine sea salt

Freshly ground black pepper

1 teaspoon coconut oil, lard, or tallow

2 large egg whites

1. Season the steaks on both sides with a pinch each of salt and pepper.

2. Heat a medium-sized cast-iron skillet over medium-high heat. Melt the oil in the hot pan, then add the steaks. Sear the steaks for 3 minutes per side, cooking them to the desired doneness. Transfer the steaks to a plate and let rest for 10 minutes. Leave the oil in the skillet and reduce the heat to medium-low.

3. Add the egg whites to the skillet and cook until firm, about 4 minutes. Remove the pan from the heat.

4. Slice the steaks and place on serving plates. Top with the egg whites. Serve immediately.

P/E ratio **7.1** • calories **208** • fat **5g** • protein **37g** • carbs **0.2g** • fiber **0g**

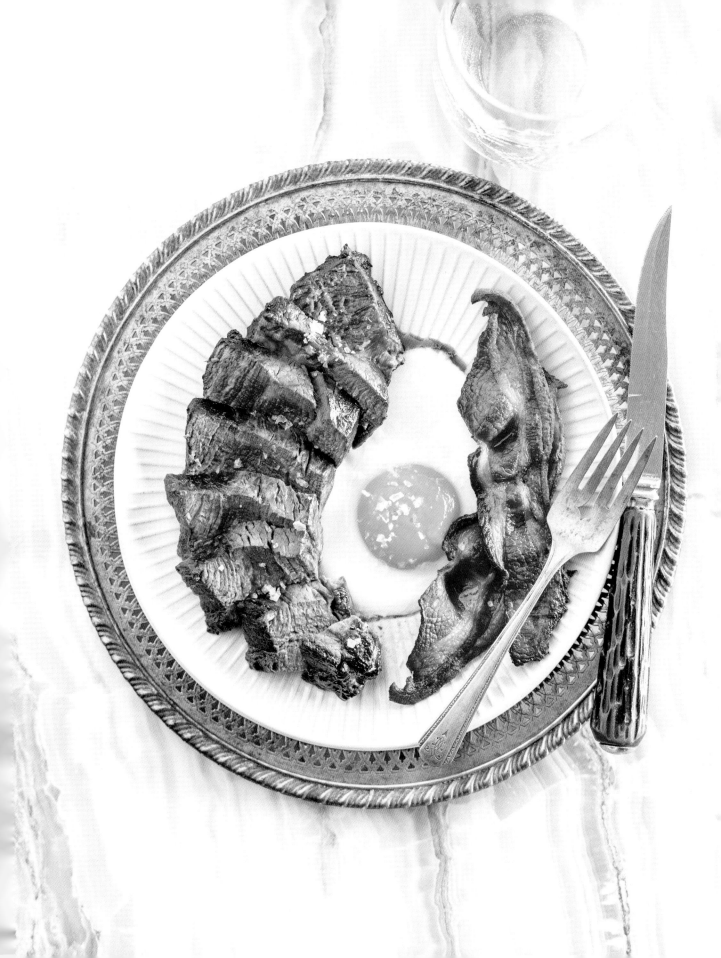

Breakfast Patties

   yield: 16 patties (2 per serving) • prep time: 5 minutes • cook time: 8 minutes per batch

For easy breakfasts on the go, make a double batch of this recipe and store the cooked patties in the refrigerator or freezer.

2 pounds 95% lean ground pork

2 teaspoons fine sea salt

2 teaspoons dried rubbed sage

½ teaspoon dried thyme leaves

1 clove garlic, minced

1 teaspoon coconut oil, lard, or tallow

1. Place the ground pork, salt, sage, thyme, and garlic in a large bowl; mix well with your hands. Divide the mixture into 16 equal portions. Form each portion into a 3-inch patty.

2. Heat the oil in a large cast-iron skillet over medium-high heat. Working in batches, cook the patties until golden brown on both sides and no longer pink inside, about 4 minutes per side. Transfer the patties to a plate and keep them warm while you cook the remaining patties. Serve warm.

3. Store leftover patties in an airtight container in the refrigerator for up to 5 days or in the freezer for up to 1 month. Reheat them in a greased cast-iron skillet over medium heat for a few minutes on each side, until warmed through.

P/E ratio **3.5** • calories **288** • fat **11g** • protein **48g** • carbs **3g** • fiber **0.2g**

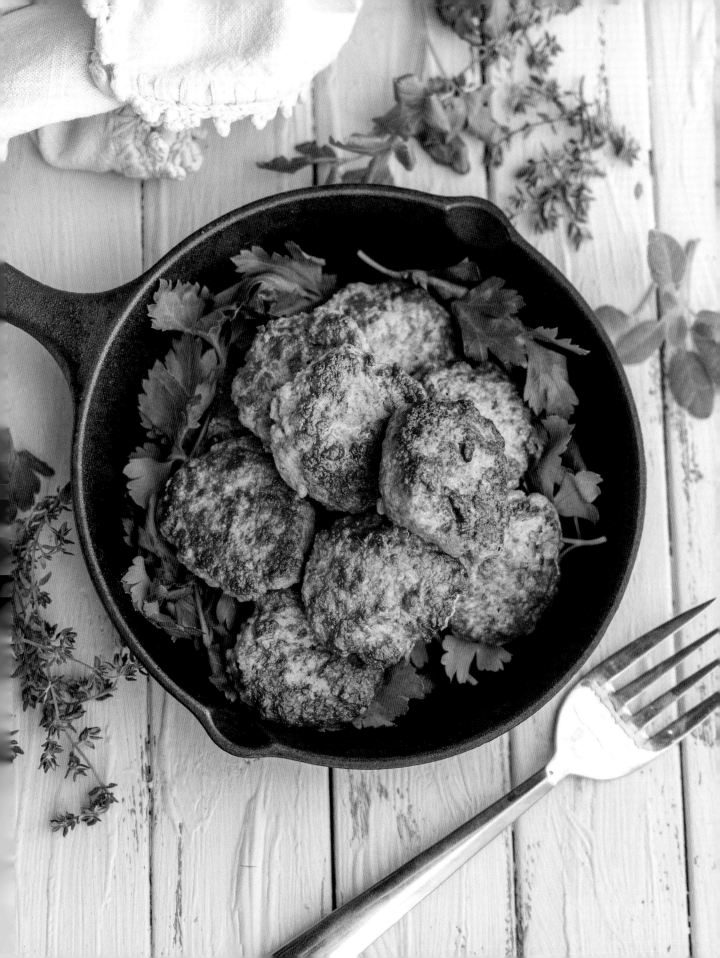

Breakfast
Sammie

  yield: 1 serving • prep time: 2 minutes (not including time to make pancakes or breakfast patty) • cook time: 2 minutes

Duck fat spray or coconut oil spray, for greasing

1 large egg white

⅛ teaspoon fine sea salt

2 Protein-Sparing Pancakes (page 66)

1 Breakfast Patty (page 62), warmed

1 slice 95% lean ham

1. Lightly grease a small nonstick skillet with duck fat spray and place it over medium-high heat.

2. Put the egg white in the skillet (you can use an egg ring if you like). Season it with the salt and cook for 1 minute; flip and cook on the other side for 1 minute. Remove the pan from the heat.

3. To assemble the sandwich, place one of the pancakes on a plate. Lay the breakfast patty, ham slice, and fried egg white on it; top with the other pancake. Serve immediately.

P/E ratio **3.8** • calories **449** • fat **14g** • protein **75g** • carbs **6g** • fiber **0.2g**

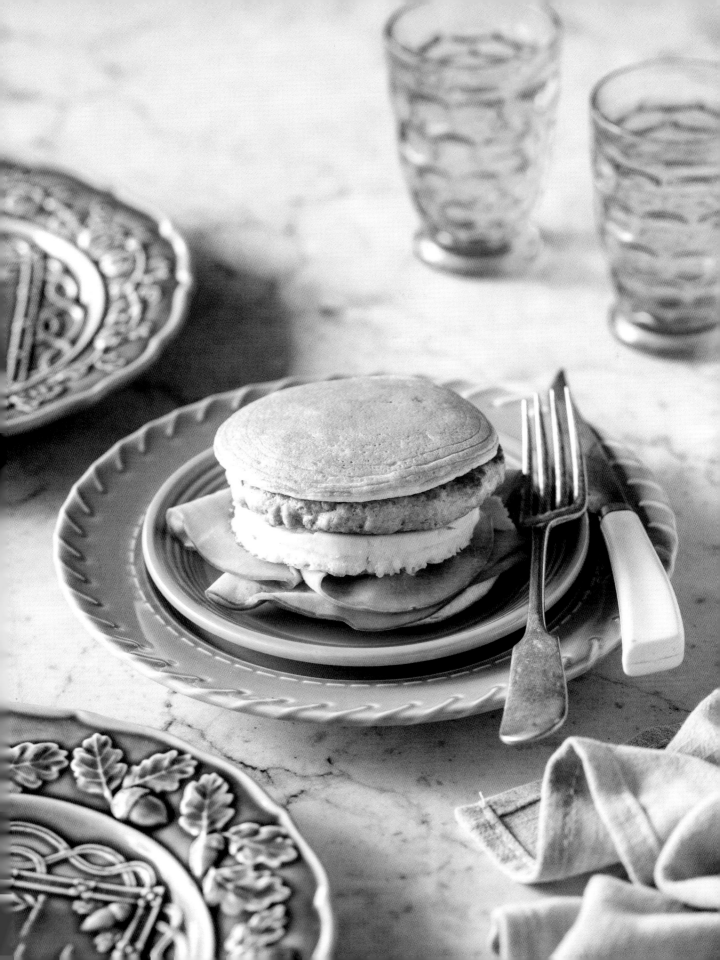

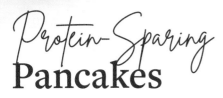

Protein-Sparing Pancakes

  yield: 2 pancakes (1 serving) • prep time: 7 minutes • cook time: 4 minutes

These pancakes are great on their own; they can also be used as buns for a Breakfast Sammie (page 64).

3 large egg whites

½ teaspoon cream of tartar

2 tablespoons unflavored egg white protein powder

1 teaspoon vanilla extract

⅛ teaspoon liquid stevia

Coconut oil spray, for greasing

1. Place the egg whites and cream of tartar in a clean, dry, cool mixing bowl. Beat with an electric hand mixer on high speed until stiff peaks form.

2. Turn the mixer down to low speed and beat in the protein powder, vanilla extract, and stevia just until combined, being careful not to deflate the whites.

3. Lightly grease a large nonstick skillet or griddle with coconut oil spray and put it over medium-high heat. Once the pan is hot, ladle half of the batter into the pan, forming a circle, about 3½ inches across. Repeat with the remaining batter. Cook until golden brown on one side, about 2 minutes; flip and cook until golden brown on the other side, about 2 minutes more.

4. Transfer the pancakes to a plate and serve warm.

P/E ratio **9.1** • calories **110** • fat **0.2g** • protein **20g** • carbs **3g** • fiber **1g**

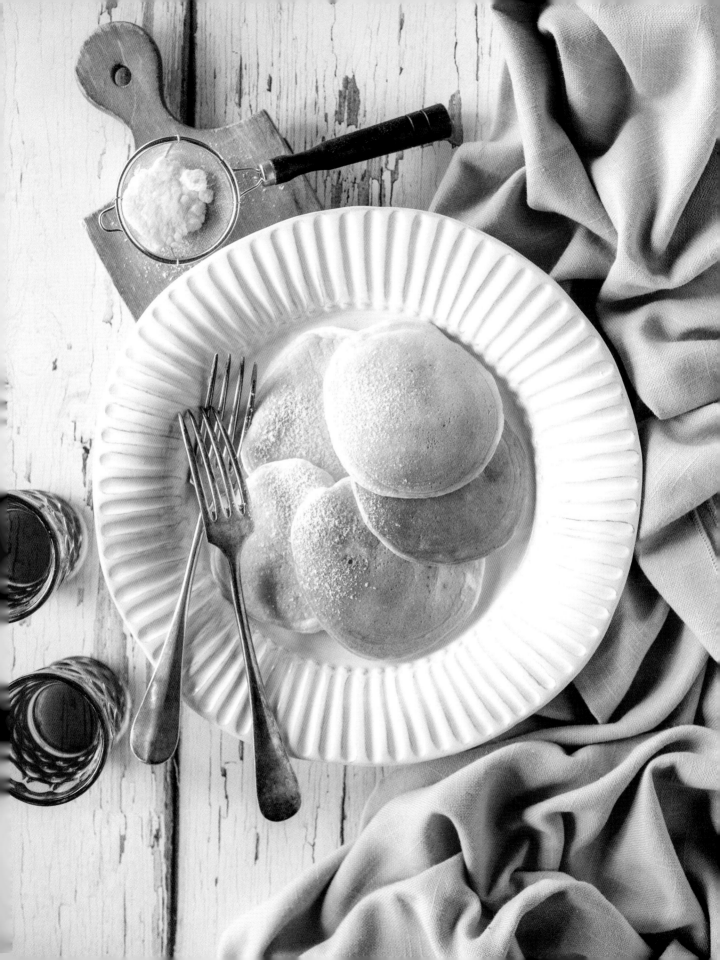

Savory Dutch Baby with Lox

  yield: 2 servings • prep time: 5 minutes • cook time: 18 minutes

6 large egg whites

¾ cup beef broth

¼ cup unflavored egg white protein powder

1 teaspoon baking powder

1 tablespoon chopped fresh dill, or 1 teaspoon dried dill weed, plus more for garnish if desired

¼ teaspoon fine sea salt

Duck fat spray or coconut oil spray, for greasing

2 ounces lox or smoked salmon

1. Place an 8-inch cast-iron skillet on a rack positioned in the middle of the oven. Set the oven to 400°F and let the skillet preheat along with the oven.

2. In a blender, blend the egg whites, broth, protein powder, baking powder, dill, and salt until foamy, about 1 minute.

3. Carefully remove the hot skillet from the oven. Grease the bottom and side of the skillet lightly with duck fat spray. Pour the batter into the skillet and return it to the oven. Bake until the pancake is puffed and golden brown, 18 to 20 minutes. Cut the pancake in half.

4. Top with the lox and garnish with more dill, if desired. Serve immediately.

P/E ratio **10.6** • calories **268** • fat **3g** • protein **53g** • carbs **2g** • fiber **0g**

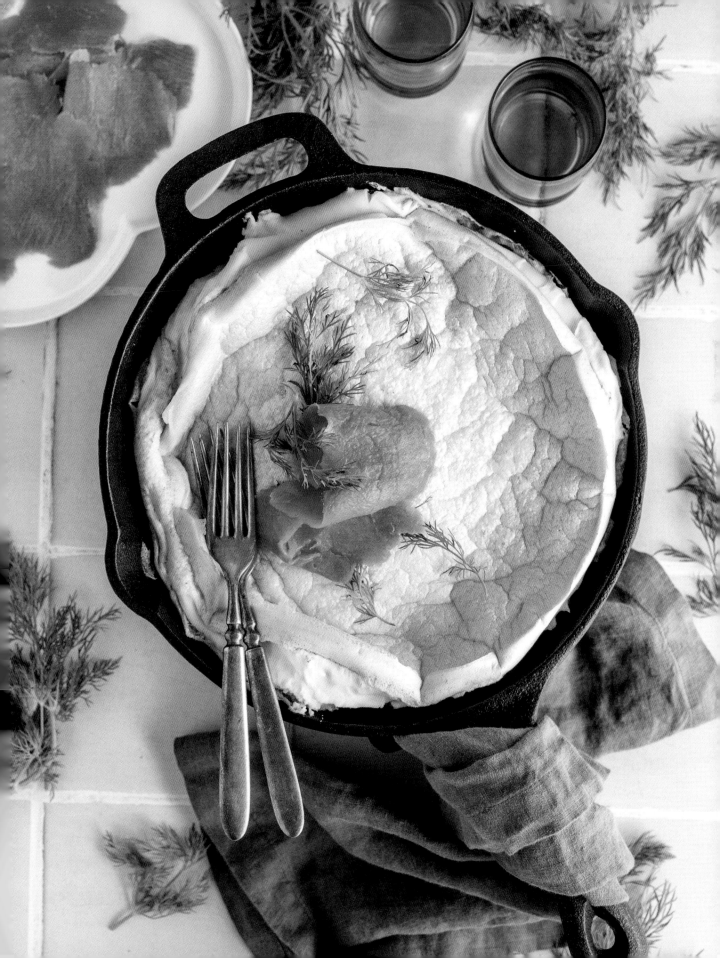

Apple
Dutch Baby

 yield: 2 servings • prep time: 5 minutes • cook time: 18 minutes

6 large egg whites

¾ cup unsweetened almond milk or cashew milk

¼ cup unflavored egg white protein powder

1 teaspoon baking powder

¼ cup confectioners'-style erythritol

2 teaspoons apple extract

¼ teaspoon fine sea salt

Coconut oil spray, for greasing

1. Place an 8-inch cast-iron skillet on a rack positioned in the middle of the oven. Set the oven to 400°F and let the skillet preheat along with the oven.

2. In a blender, blend the egg whites, milk, protein powder, baking powder, sweetener, apple extract, and salt until foamy, about 1 minute.

3. Carefully remove the hot skillet from the oven. Grease the bottom and side of the pan lightly with coconut oil spray. Pour the batter into the skillet and return it to the oven. Bake until the pancake is puffed and golden brown, 18 to 20 minutes.

4. Cut the pancake in half and serve immediately.

P/E ratio **8.9** • calories **212** • fat **2g** • protein **41g** • carbs **3g** • fiber **0.4g**

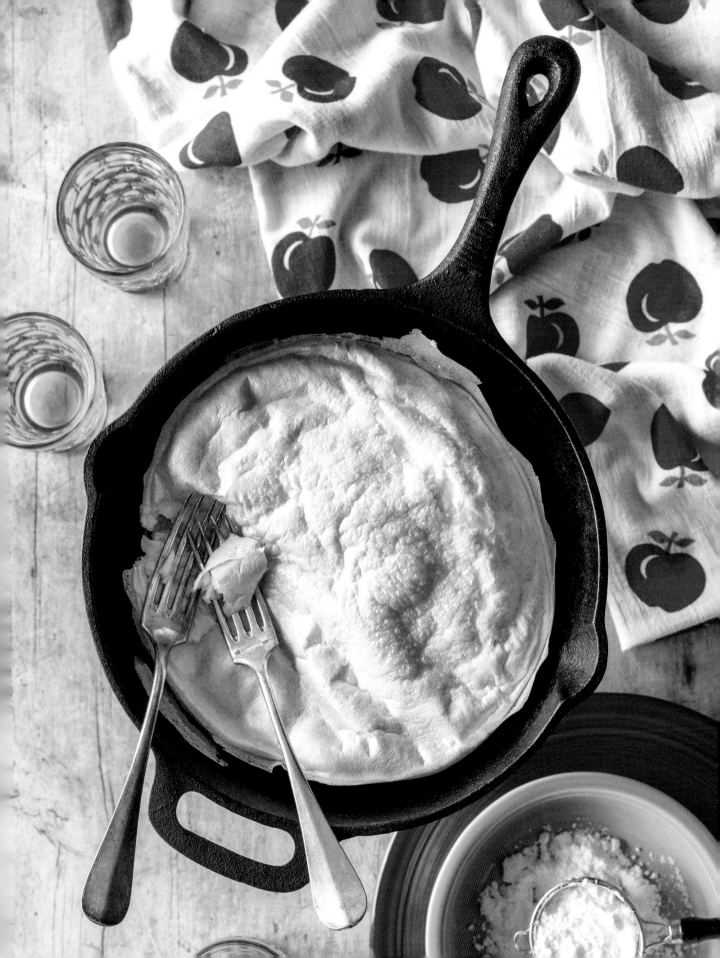

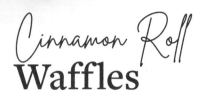

Cinnamon Roll Waffles

  yield: 2 waffles (1 serving) • prep time: 4 minutes (not including time to make pudding) • cook time: 4 minutes

These waffles will make you feel like you're eating a cinnamon roll! They're also quick and easy to make. The only piece of equipment you need is a mini waffle maker.

2 large egg whites

2 tablespoons vanilla-flavored or unflavored egg white protein powder

2 teaspoons ground cinnamon, plus more for sprinkling if desired

½ teaspoon maple extract (optional)

½ cup French Vanilla Breakfast Pudding (page 84)

Coconut oil spray, for greasing

Special Equipment:

Mini waffle maker

1. Preheat a mini waffle maker.

2. Put the egg whites in a medium-sized bowl and beat with an electric hand mixer on high speed until stiff peaks form. Add the protein powder, cinnamon, and maple extract, if using, and beat on low until just combined, being careful not to deflate the whites.

3. Spray the waffle maker with coconut oil spray. Spoon half of the batter into the center. Cook until firm and golden brown, 2 to 3 minutes. Remove the waffle to a serving plate and repeat with the remaining batter.

4. Top each waffle with ¼ cup of the pudding and sprinkle with cinnamon. Serve immediately.

P/E ratio **4.8** • calories **136** • fat **1g** • protein **24g** • carbs **5g** • fiber **2g**

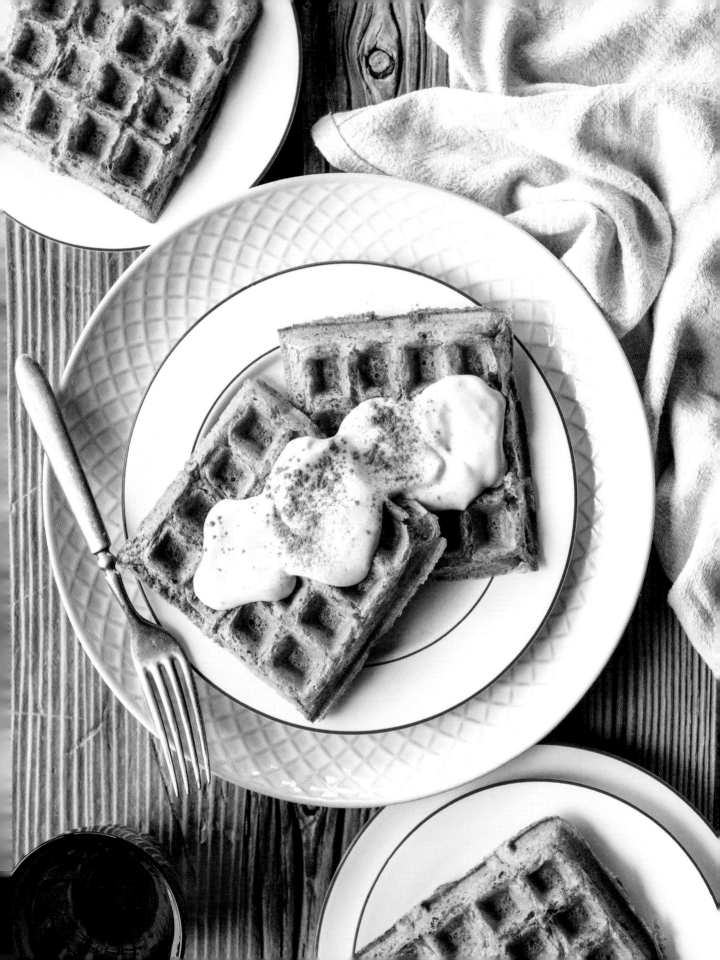

Classic
French Toast

  yield: 4 slices (2 per serving) • prep time: 2 minutes (not including time to make bread) • cook time: 4 minutes

2 large egg whites

½ teaspoon vanilla extract

¼ teaspoon ground cinnamon, plus more for sprinkling

⅛ teaspoon fine sea salt

⅛ teaspoon maple-flavored liquid stevia

Coconut oil spray, for greasing

4 slices Protein-Sparing Bread or Cinnamon Protein-Sparing Bread (page 270)

1. In a medium-sized shallow dish, beat the egg whites, vanilla extract, cinnamon, salt, and stevia with a fork just until combined.

2. Lightly grease a large nonstick skillet with coconut oil spray and place it over medium-high heat.

3. Dip the bread in the egg white mixture, coating both sides. Carefully lay the bread in the hot skillet.

4. Cook until golden brown on one side, about 2 minutes; flip and cook until golden brown on the other side, about 2 minutes more.

5. Sprinkle with more cinnamon and serve warm.

P/E ratio **5.0** • calories **210** • fat **5g** • protein **35g** • carbs **3g** • fiber **1g**

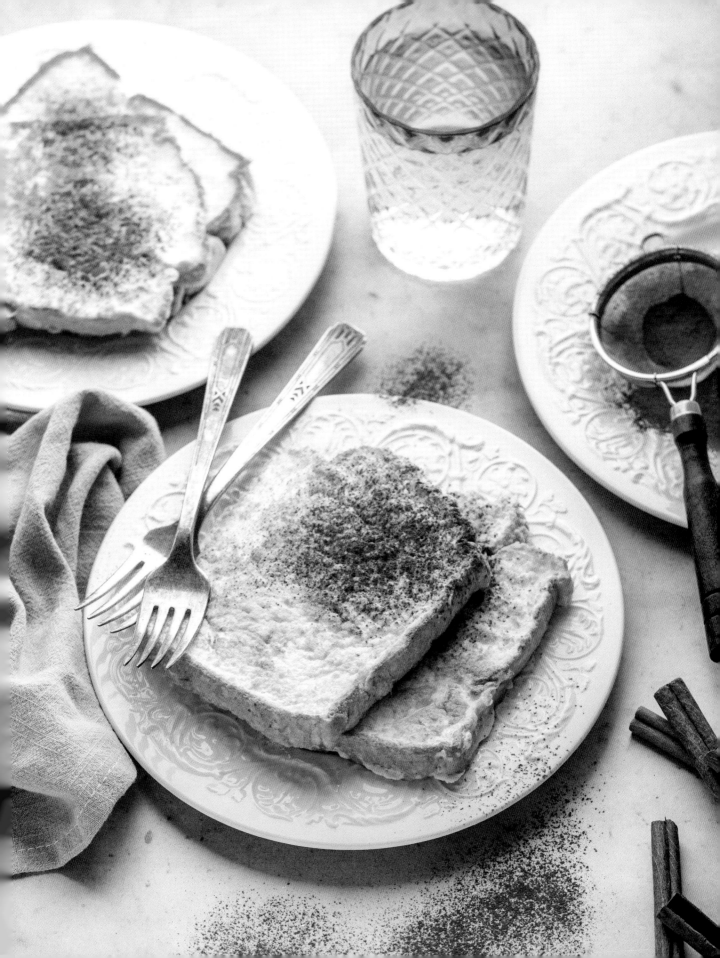

Strawberry Angel Food French Toast

  yield: 2 slices (1 serving) • prep time: 5 minutes (not including time to make cake) • cook time: 4 minutes

2 large egg whites

½ teaspoon vanilla extract

⅛ teaspoon fine sea salt

⅛ teaspoon liquid stevia

Coconut oil spray, for greasing

2 slices Strawberry Angel Food Cake (page 246)

1. In a medium-sized shallow dish, beat the egg whites, vanilla extract, salt, and stevia with a fork just until combined.

2. Lightly grease a medium-sized nonstick skillet with coconut oil spray and place it over medium-high heat.

3. Dip the cake slices into the egg white mixture, coating both sides. Carefully lay the cake in the hot skillet.

4. Cook until golden brown on one side, about 2 minutes; flip and cook until golden brown on the other side, about 2 minutes more.

5. Transfer to a serving plate and serve warm.

P/E ratio **8.2** • calories **136** • fat **0.3g** • protein **27g** • carbs **3g** • fiber **0g**

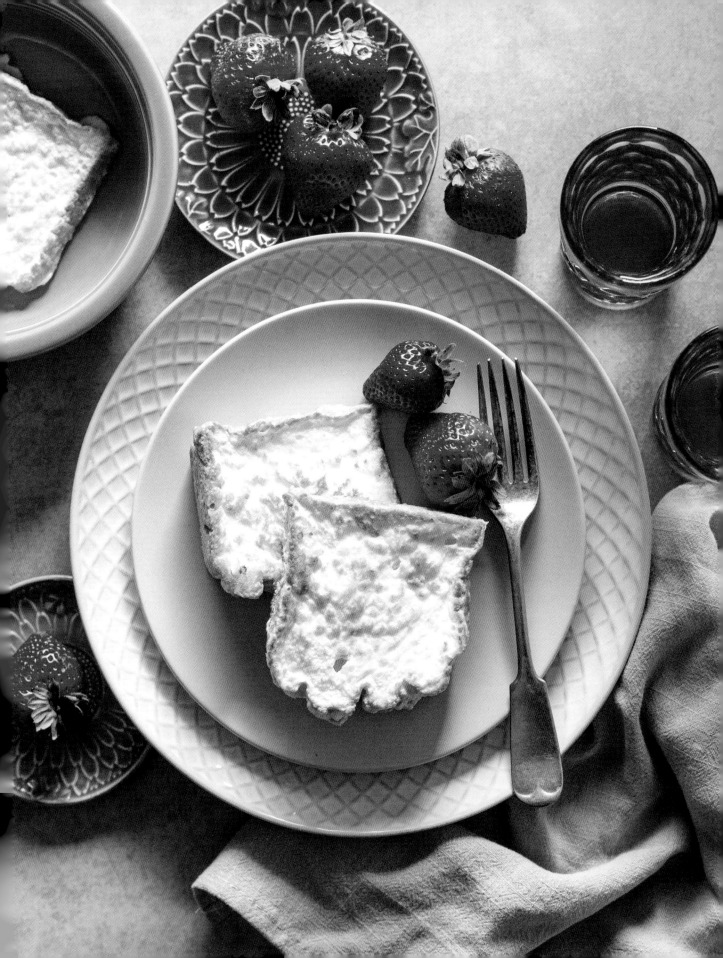

Minute
Breakfast Muffins

   yield: 6 muffins (3 per serving) • prep time: 2 minutes • cook time: 1 minute

These muffins live up to their name: just one minute in the microwave, and breakfast is ready!

6 (4-inch) slices 95% lean ham

12 large egg whites

½ teaspoon fine sea salt

¼ teaspoon freshly ground black pepper

2 tablespoons chopped fresh basil leaves, for garnish

1. Line each of six 4-ounce ramekins or 6 wells of a microwave-safe muffin pan with a slice of ham. Put 2 egg whites in each ham cup. Season with the salt and pepper.

2. Microwave on high until the egg whites are set, about 1 minute.

3. Garnish with the basil and serve immediately.

P/E ratio **3.2** • calories **207** • fat **8g** • protein **31g** • carbs **2g** • fiber **0.2g**

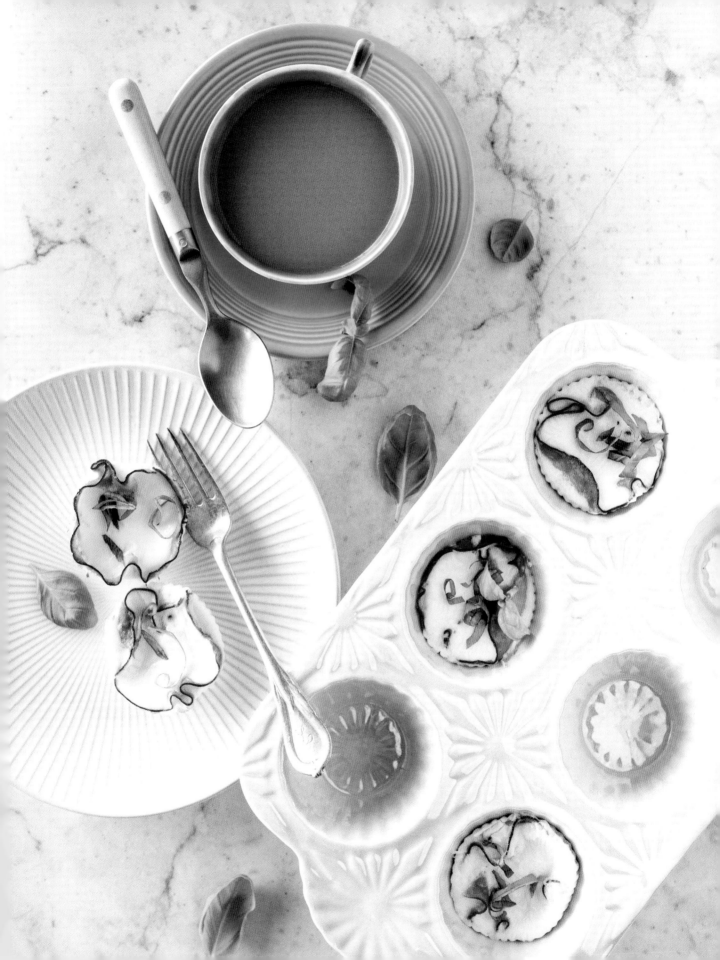

French Toast Porridge

 yield: 1 serving • prep time: 5 minutes • cook time: 4 minutes

8 large egg whites

⅔ cup unsweetened almond milk or cashew milk, plus more for serving if desired

¼ cup confectioners'-style erythritol

1 teaspoon maple extract

½ teaspoon fine sea salt

1 teaspoon coconut oil (preferably butter-flavored)

Ground cinnamon, for sprinkling

1. In a medium-sized bowl, whisk together the egg whites, milk, sweetener, maple extract, and salt until well combined.

2. In a medium-sized saucepan, melt the oil over medium heat. Add the egg white mixture and whisk constantly until the mixture thickens and small curds form, about 4 minutes. Remove the pan from the heat.

3. Transfer the porridge to a serving bowl. Sprinkle with cinnamon and top with more milk, if desired. Serve warm.

P/E ratio **3.4** • calories **195** • fat **7g** • protein **29g** • carbs **2g** • fiber **0.4g**

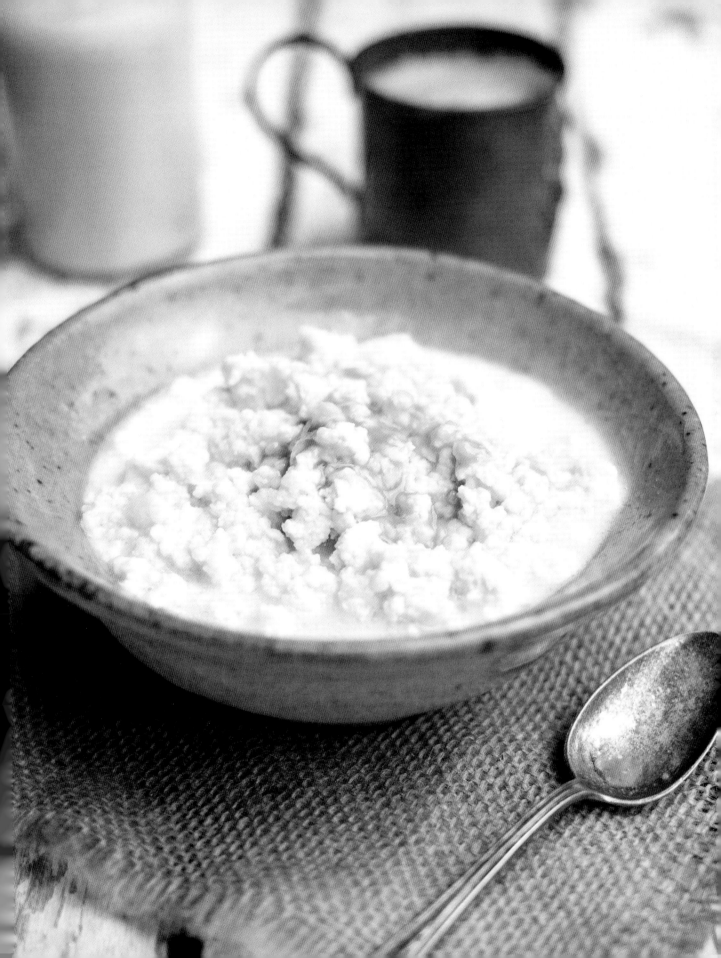

Chocolate
Hot Breakfast Cereal

 yield: 1 serving • prep time: 4 minutes • cook time: 4 minutes

This recipe is my protein-sparing copycat of the chocolate-flavored Malt-O-Meal cereal that I grew up eating. It's better than the original, if I do say so myself!

8 large egg whites

⅔ cup unsweetened almond milk or cashew milk, plus more for serving if desired

½ teaspoon stevia glycerite, or a few drops liquid stevia

4 teaspoons vanilla extract

1 tablespoon unsweetened cocoa powder

½ teaspoon fine sea salt

1 teaspoon coconut oil (preferably butter-flavored)

1. In a medium-sized bowl, whisk together the egg whites, milk, stevia, vanilla extract, cocoa powder, and salt until well combined.

2. In a medium-sized saucepan, melt the oil over medium heat. Add the egg white mixture and whisk constantly until the mixture thickens and small curds form, about 4 minutes. Remove the pan from the heat.

3. Transfer the cereal to a serving bowl. Top with more milk, if desired, and serve warm.

P/E ratio **2.3** • calories **262** • fat **8g** • protein **30g** • carbs **6g** • fiber **1g**

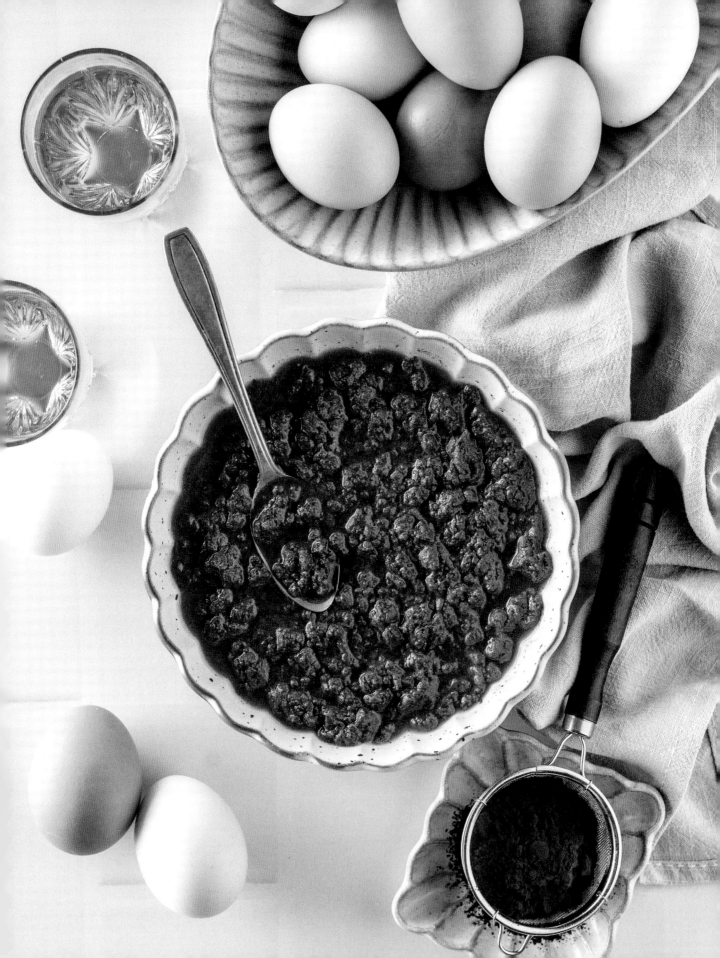

Chocolate
Breakfast Pudding

 yield: 2 servings • prep time: 5 minutes, plus time to chill

10 large hard-boiled egg whites, or 1¼ cups 100% liquid egg whites, lightly scrambled

1 cup unsweetened almond milk or cashew milk

¼ cup confectioners'-style erythritol, or more to taste

2½ tablespoons unsweetened cocoa powder

2 teaspoons vanilla extract

½ teaspoon ground cinnamon

⅛ teaspoon fine sea salt

1. Place all of the ingredients in a blender and puree until smooth. Taste and add more sweetener if desired.

2. Divide the pudding between two serving glasses and refrigerate until well chilled before serving.

Variations:

- Banana Breakfast Pudding: Omit the cocoa powder and replace the vanilla extract with banana extract.

- Black Forest Breakfast Pudding: Increase the cocoa powder to ¼ cup and replace the vanilla extract with cherry extract.

- Butterscotch Breakfast Pudding: Omit the cocoa powder and replace the vanilla extract with 1 tablespoon butterscotch extract.

- French Toast Breakfast Pudding: Omit the cocoa powder, add 1½ teaspoons ground cinnamon, and replace the vanilla extract with maple extract.

- French Vanilla Breakfast Pudding: Omit the cocoa powder.

- Key Lime Breakfast Pudding: Omit the cocoa powder and replace the vanilla extract with 4 teaspoons key lime extract.

- Lemon Breakfast Pudding: Omit the cocoa powder and replace the vanilla extract with 4 teaspoons lemon extract.

P/E ratio **5.3** • calories **113** • fat **2g** • protein **19g** • carbs **2g** • fiber **0.4g**

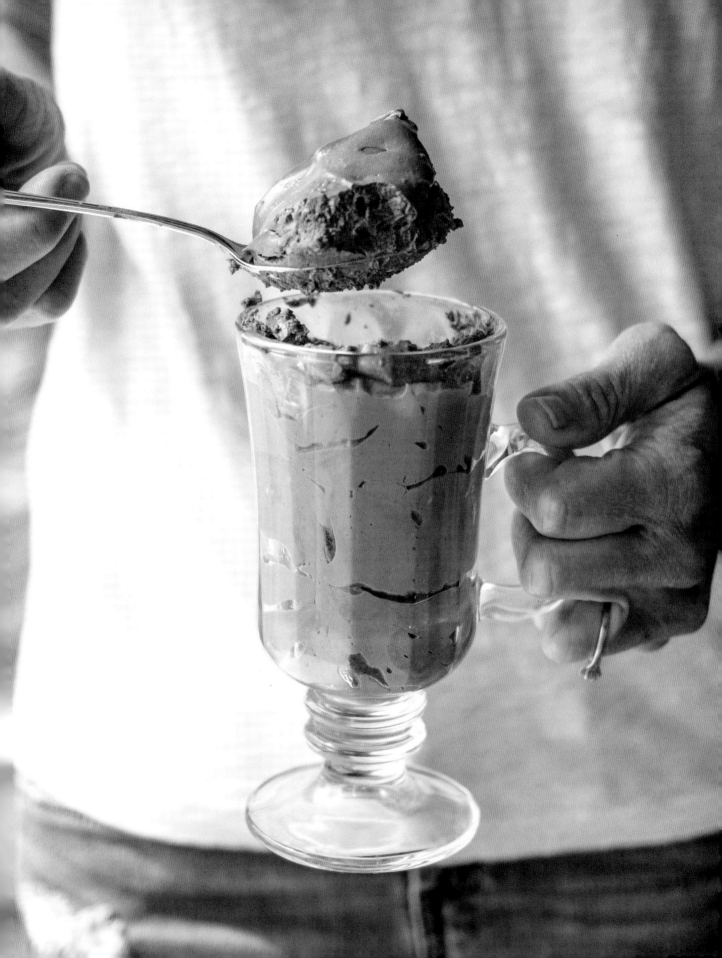

Strawberry Shake

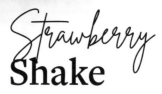

  yield: 1 serving • prep time: 2 minutes

1 cup unsweetened almond milk or cashew milk

½ cup vanilla-flavored beef protein powder or unflavored egg white protein powder

1 teaspoon strawberry extract

⅛ teaspoon strawberry-flavored liquid stevia

Put all of the ingredients in a blender and puree until smooth. Serve immediately.

P/E ratio **9.8** • calories **203** • fat **3g** • protein **39g** • carbs **2g** • fiber **1g**

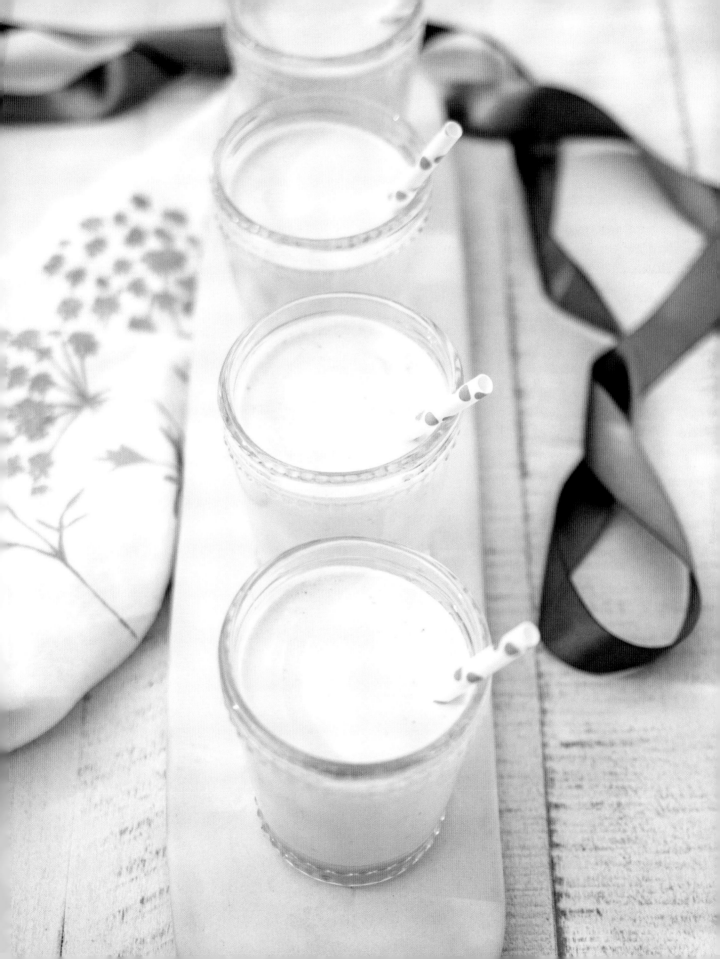

Orange Creamsicle Smoothie

 yield: 2 servings • prep time: 5 minutes, plus time to chill overnight

This smoothie is best enjoyed chilled, so make it the night before (or up to four days in advance) and serve it cold for breakfast.

10 large hard-boiled egg whites, or 1¼ cups 100% liquid egg whites, lightly scrambled

1½ cups unsweetened almond milk or cashew milk

¼ cup confectioners'-style erythritol, or more to taste

2 teaspoons orange extract

⅛ teaspoon orange-flavored liquid stevia

⅛ teaspoon fine sea salt

1. Put all of the ingredients in a blender and puree until smooth. Taste and add more sweetener if desired.

2. Transfer to an airtight container and chill overnight before pouring into glasses and serving.

P/E ratio **6.3** • calories **215** • fat **4g** • protein **38g** • carbs **3g** • fiber **1g**

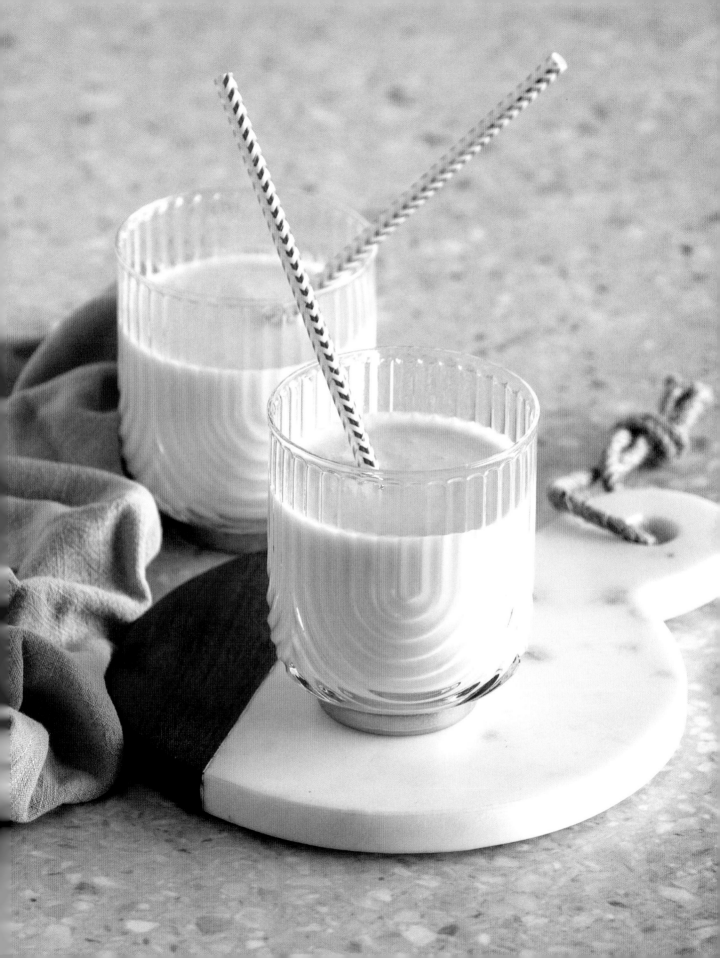

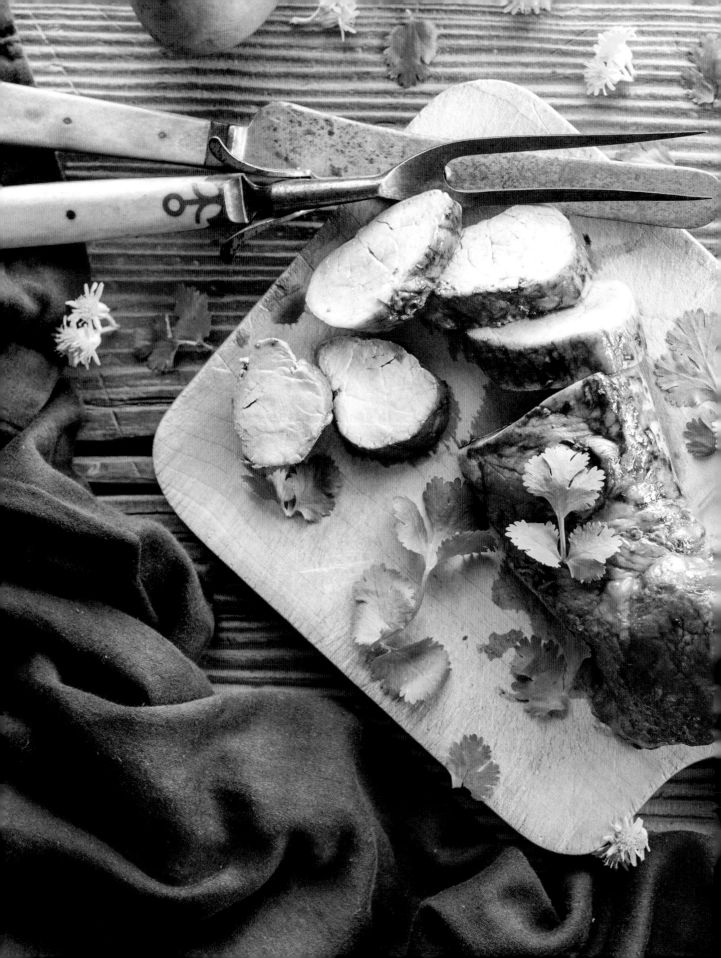

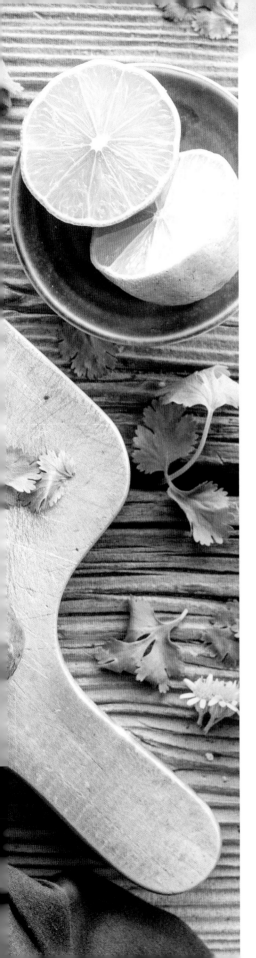

chapter 2

Main Dishes
Beef & Pork

Hamburger Patties with Mustard / 92

Slow Cooker Shredded Pork Loin / 94

Baked Pork Tenderloins / 96

Pork Chops with Dijon Vinaigrette / 98

Grilled Filet Mignons with
Truffle Mustard Sauce / 100

BBQ Pork Chops / 102

Grilled Flank Steak with Chimichurri Sauce / 104

BBQ Meatloaf / 106

Asian-Style Meatballs / 108

Sweet and Sour Pork Chops / 110

Garlic-Thyme Pork Tenderloins / 112

BBQ Meatballs / 114

Grilled Pork Chops with
Truffle Mustard Sauce / 116

Hamburger Patties
with Mustard

   yield: 8 patties (4 per serving) • prep time: 8 minutes • cook time: 6 minutes

I like to serve these patties with smoked venison jerky for extra protein and the smoky bacon flavor.

Duck fat or coconut oil, for greasing

1 pound 95% lean ground beef

2½ teaspoons fine sea salt

1½ teaspoons freshly ground black pepper

½ cup prepared yellow mustard or Carolina BBQ Sauce (page 267), for serving

Venison Jerky (page 222), for serving (optional)

1. Lightly grease the grates of a grill with duck fat. Heat the grill to medium heat.

2. Divide the ground beef into 8 equal portions. Form each portion into a patty, about ½ inch thick. Season on both sides with the salt and pepper.

3. Grill on one side for 3 minutes. Flip and cook the other side until no longer pink inside, about 3 minutes more.

4. Serve with the mustard and, if desired, the jerky on the side.

P/E ratio **4.2** • calories **312** • fat **11g** • protein **49g** • carbs **1g** • fiber **0.4g**

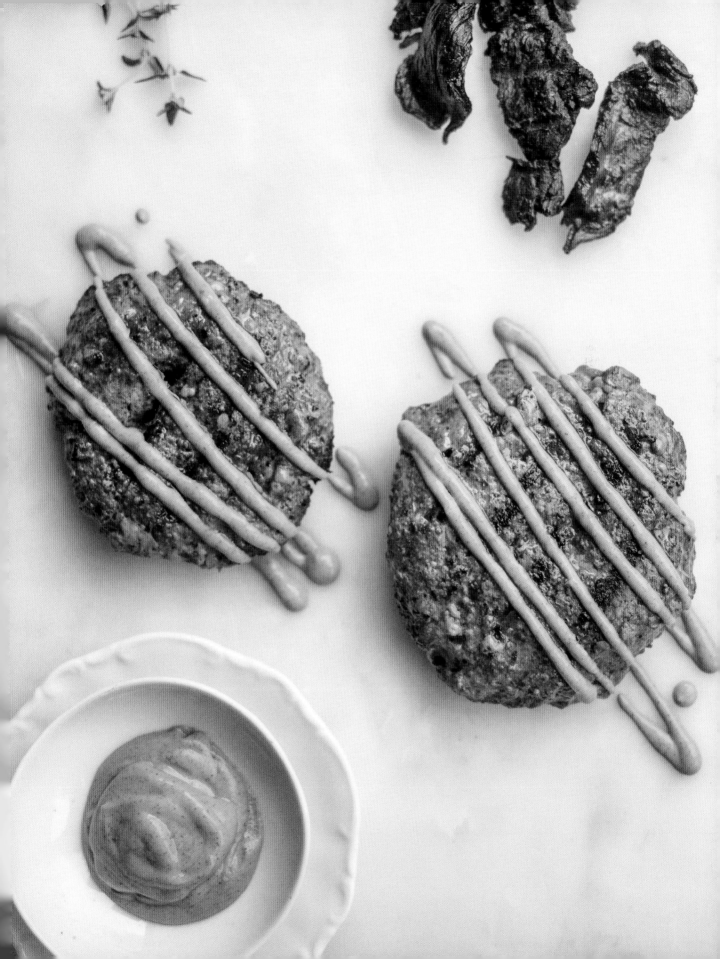

Slow Cooker
Shredded Pork Loin

   yield: 8 servings • prep time: 5 minutes • cook time: 8 hours

4 pounds boneless pork loin

5 cloves garlic, halved lengthwise

2 cups chicken broth

½ cup tomato sauce

¼ cup diced yellow onions

2 teaspoons liquid smoke

2 tablespoons smoked paprika

1½ teaspoons chili powder

1 teaspoon fine sea salt

1 teaspoon freshly ground black pepper

1. Using the tip of a paring knife, make 10 pockets all over the pork loin. Tuck a garlic clove half into each pocket.

2. Place the pork loin in a 6-quart slow cooker. Add the remaining ingredients. Cover and cook on low for 8 hours, or until the meat is tender and the internal temperature reaches 145°F.

3. Shred the pork with two forks and mix it well with the juice before serving.

4. Store leftover pork in an airtight container in the refrigerator for up to 5 days. To reheat, place in a saucepan over medium heat for 5 minutes, or until warmed through.

note: *To cook the pork in an Instant Pot, place the garlic-studded roast in the Instant Pot and add the rest of the ingredients. Seal and press Manual to cook for 1 hour. Once finished, press Natural Release.*

P/E ratio **3.8** • calories **313** • fat **10g** • protein **49g** • carbs **5g** • fiber **2g**

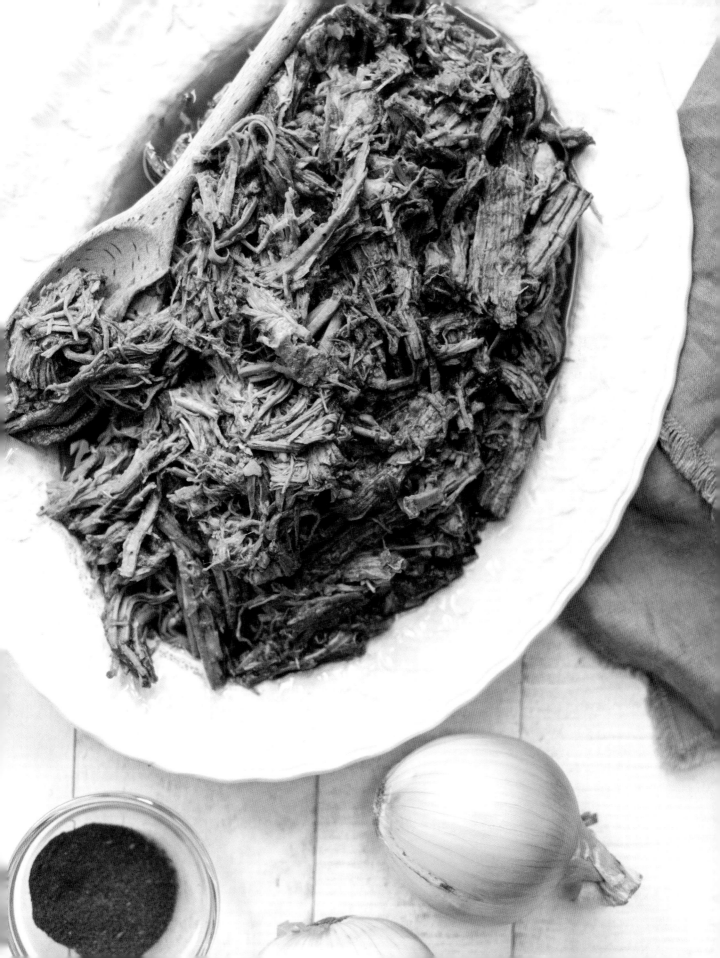

Baked
Pork Tenderloins

   yield: 8 servings • prep time: 5 minutes, plus 10 minutes to rest • cook time: 40 minutes

I like purchasing packages of two small tenderloins rather than one large tenderloin. Smaller tenderloins cook faster, which gets dinner on the table that much quicker!

2 (2-pound) pork tenderloins

8 cloves garlic, halved lengthwise

2 tablespoons wheat-free tamari

2 tablespoons lime juice

1 tablespoon peeled and grated fresh ginger

⅛ teaspoon liquid stevia

⅛ teaspoon orange extract (optional)

For Garnish (optional):

Chopped fresh cilantro leaves

Lime slices

1. Preheat the oven to 350°F. Line a 9 by 13-inch baking dish with parchment paper.

2. Place the pork tenderloins in the prepared baking dish. Using the tip of a paring knife, make 8 pockets all over each tenderloin. Tuck a garlic clove half into each pocket.

3. In a small bowl, stir the tamari, lime juice, ginger, stevia, and extract, if using, until well combined. Pour the mixture over the pork.

4. Bake until the internal temperature of the pork reaches 145°F, about 40 minutes. Place the pork on a cutting board to rest for 10 minutes.

5. Cut the pork into ½-inch slices and arrange on a platter. Pour the juices from the baking dish over them. Garnish with cilantro and/or lime slices, if desired.

P/E ratio **3.2** • calories **324** • fat **13g** • protein **47g** • carbs **2g** • fiber **0.1g**

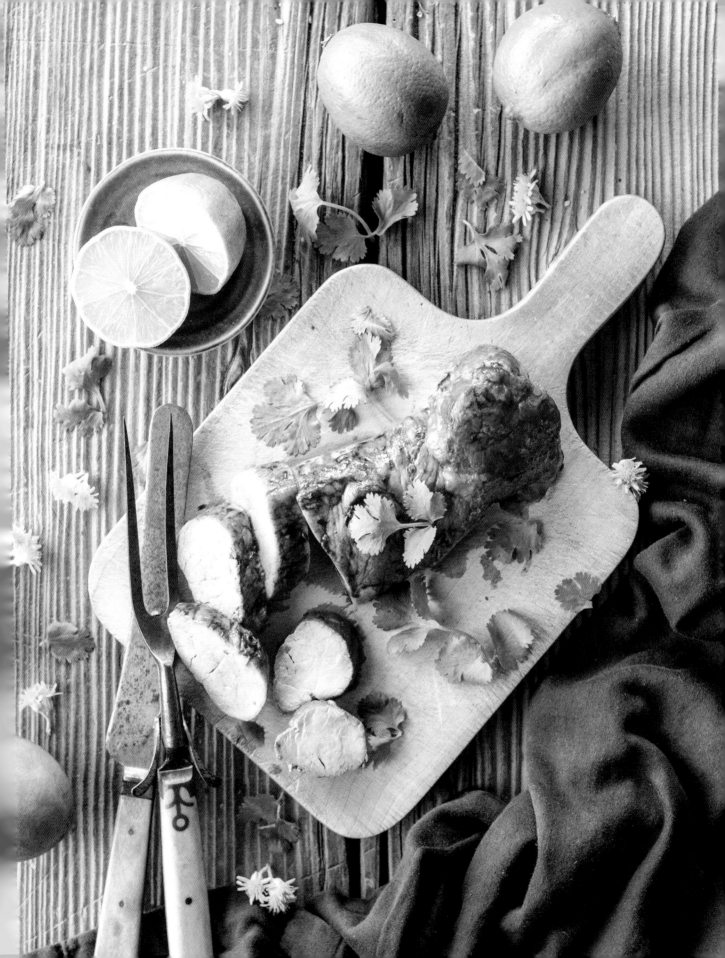

Pork Chops
with Dijon Vinaigrette

   yield: 4 servings • prep time: 10 minutes (not including time to make vinaigrette) • cook time: 7 minutes

1 tablespoon coconut oil, lard, or tallow

4 (5-ounce) bone-in pork chops, visible fat removed

Fine sea salt and freshly ground black pepper

½ cup Dijon Vinaigrette (page 266)

3 teaspoons fresh thyme leaves, plus more for garnish (optional)

1. Heat the oil in a large cast-iron skillet over medium-high heat.

2. Pat the pork chops dry with paper towels and season both sides liberally with salt and pepper. When the oil is hot, cook the chops until golden brown on one side, about 3 minutes; flip and continue to cook until the other side is golden brown and the internal temperature reaches 145°F, about 3 minutes more. (Do not overcrowd the pan; if necessary, cook the chops in batches.)

3. Remove the chops from the skillet and set aside to rest, keeping the pan on the heat. Add the vinaigrette to the drippings in the skillet and whisk slowly to combine. Bring to a simmer and reduce the liquid a little, about 1 minute, then remove the pan from the heat. Stir in the thyme, if using, and season with more salt and pepper if needed.

4. Plate the chops and spoon the pan sauce over them. Garnish with additional thyme, if desired.

P/E ratio **1.5** • calories **381** • fat **23g** • protein **36g** • carbs **2g** • fiber **0.2g**

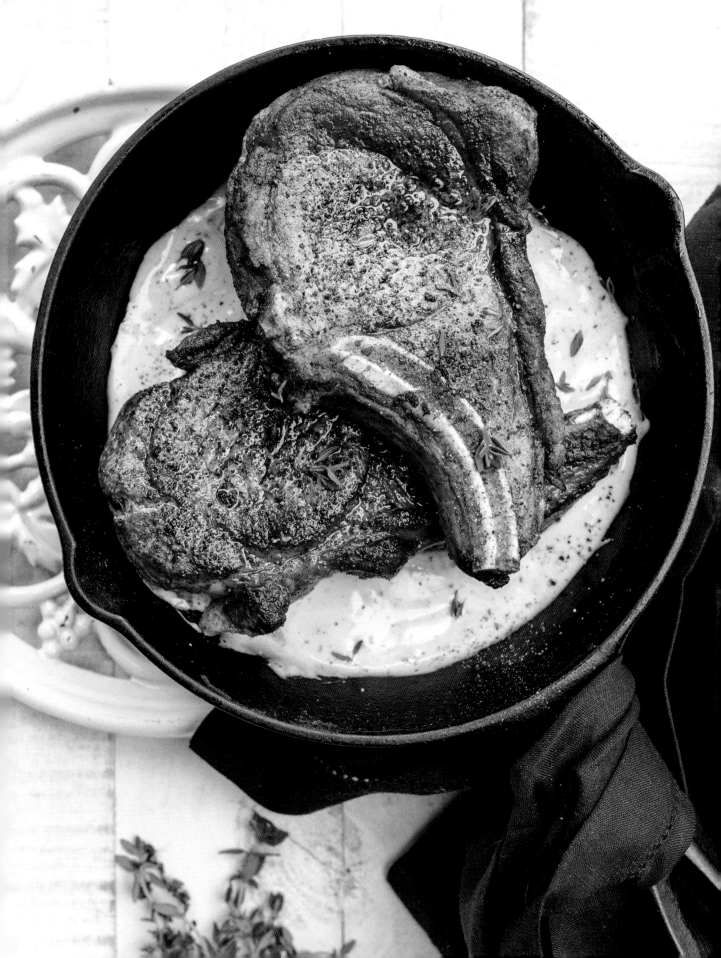

Grilled Filet Mignons
with Truffle Mustard Sauce

   yield: 1 serving • prep time: 8 minutes, plus 25 minutes to rest (not including time to make sauce) • cook time: 15 minutes

This sauce is a flavor bomb! In addition to steaks, it's delicious on pork chops, burgers, chicken, and more. Truffles are edible fungi that have an intense flavor and scent; a little goes a long way. For this sauce, I use jarred black truffles preserved in olive oil, which you can find online. You can also use truffle salt in place of sea salt if you can't find black truffles.

2 (3-ounce) filet mignons

Fine sea salt and freshly ground black pepper

Duck fat or coconut oil, for greasing

Fresh parsley leaves, for garnish (optional)

Truffle Mustard Sauce (*makes ¼ cup*):

¼ cup Dijon mustard or prepared yellow mustard

¼ teaspoon minced black truffle

⅛ teaspoon fine sea salt

1. Season the filets well on all sides with salt and pepper. Let sit at room temperature for 15 minutes.

2. Lightly grease the grates of a grill with duck fat. Heat the grill to medium-high heat. Once hot, grill the steaks for 4 minutes per side for medium-rare. Set the steaks aside to rest for 10 minutes.

3. Make the sauce: Put the mustard, truffle, and salt in a small bowl and stir well to combine.

4. Cut the steaks into slices. Garnish with parsley, if desired, and serve with 1 tablespoon of the sauce.

5. Store leftover sauce in a jar in the refrigerator for up to 1 week.

P/E ratio **3.2** • calories **253** • fat **11g** • protein **35g** • carbs **1g** • fiber **1g**

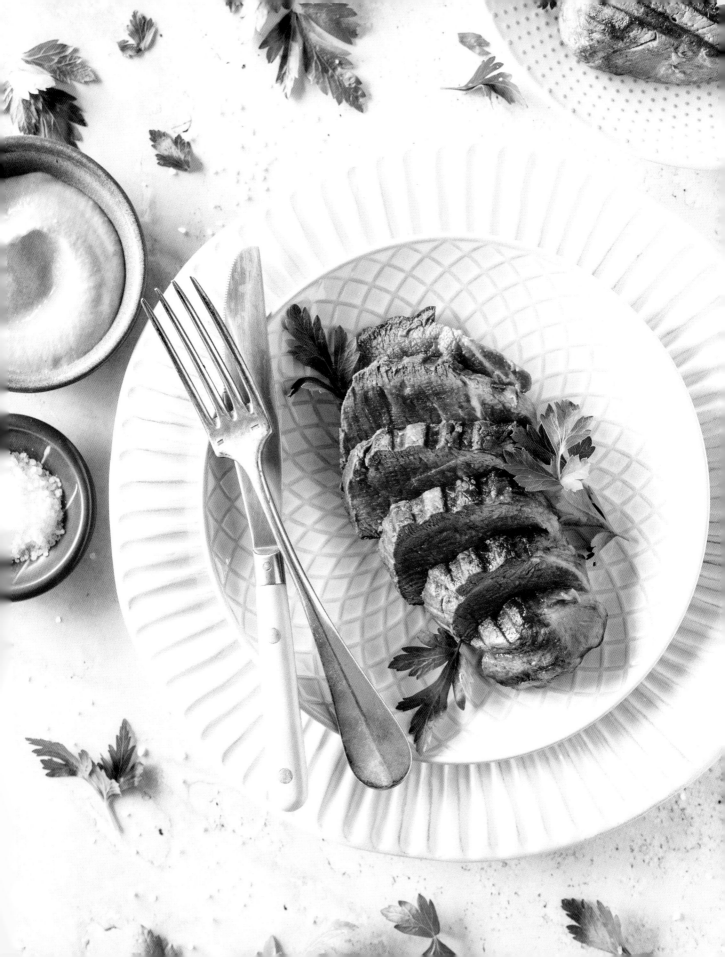

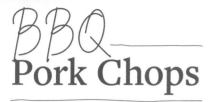

BBQ
Pork Chops

   yield: 4 servings • prep time: 5 minutes (not including time to make BBQ sauce) • cook time: 6 minutes

Duck fat or coconut oil, for greasing

4 (5-ounce) bone-in pork chops, visible fat removed

Fine sea salt and freshly ground black pepper

BBQ Sauce (*makes 1½ cups*):

1 cup tomato sauce

2 tablespoons coconut vinegar or apple cider vinegar

1½ teaspoons liquid smoke

⅛ teaspoon liquid stevia, or more to taste

½ teaspoon garlic powder

½ teaspoon onion powder

½ teaspoon freshly ground black pepper

Pinch of fine sea salt

1. Lightly grease the grates of a grill with duck fat. Heat the grill to medium-high heat.

2. Pat the pork chops dry with paper towels and season both sides liberally with salt and pepper. Grill the chops until golden brown on one side, about 3 minutes; flip and grill until the internal temperature reaches 145°F, about 3 minutes more.

3. Meanwhile, make the sauce: In a large bowl, whisk all of the ingredients until well combined. Taste and add more sweetener if needed.

4. Brush the chops with ½ cup of the BBQ sauce and grill for a few seconds. Brush the other side and grill for a few more seconds. Remove from the grill and serve with extra sauce.

5. Store leftover BBQ sauce in a jar in the refrigerator for up to a week.

P/E ratio **1.4** • calories **301** • fat **19g** • protein **28g** • carbs **2g** • fiber **1g**

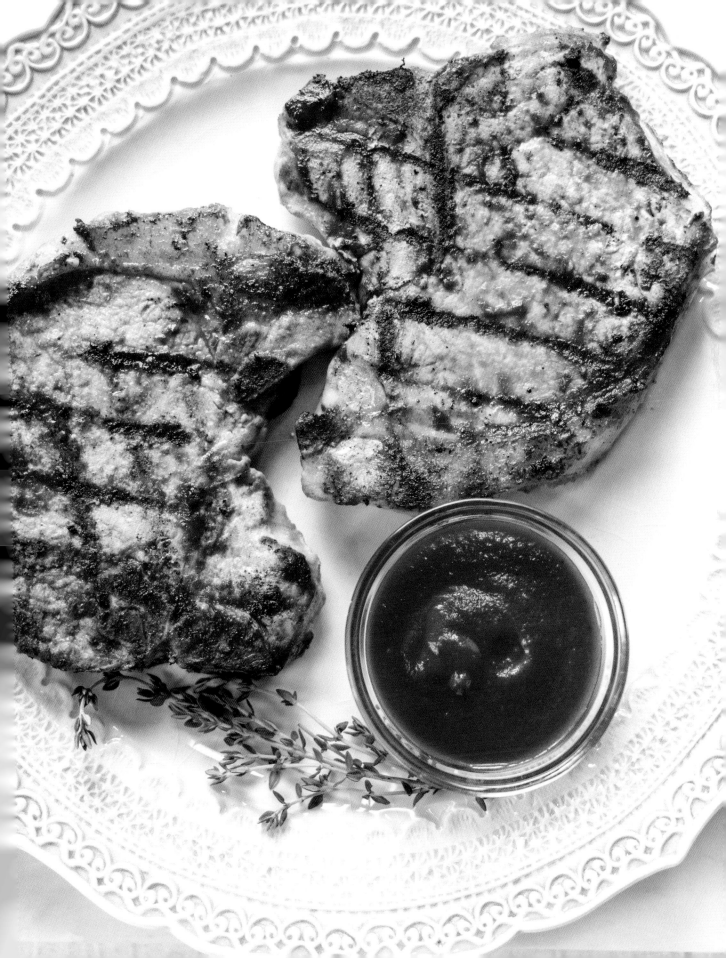

Grilled Flank Steak
with Chimichurri Sauce

   yield: 6 servings • prep time: 15 minutes, plus 2 hours to marinate and 5 minutes to rest (not including time to make sauce) • cook time: 6 minutes

1 (1½-pound) flank steak

¼ cup lime juice

2 cloves garlic, minced

1 tablespoon fine sea salt

1½ teaspoons freshly ground black pepper

1 teaspoon ground dried oregano

1 teaspoon ground dried thyme

Duck fat or coconut oil, for greasing

For Serving:

¾ cup Chimichurri Sauce (page 260)

6 lime wedges

1. Place two layers of plastic wrap on a large work surface and lay the flank steak on it. Cover the steak with additional plastic wrap. Using a meat mallet, pound the steak on both sides until it is an even ¼ inch thick.

2. In a large, deep bowl, mix together the lime juice, garlic, salt, pepper, oregano, and thyme. Put the steak in the bowl and turn to coat. Cover the bowl and place in the refrigerator to marinate for at least 2 hours or overnight.

3. About 45 minutes before you're ready to grill the steak, remove it from the marinade and allow it to come to room temperature.

4. Lightly grease the grates of a grill with duck fat. Heat the grill to medium-high heat.

5. When the grill is hot, grill the steak for 3 to 4 minutes per side for medium-rare, or to your preferred doneness. (Give the steak a quarter turn after 1½ minutes to form crisscross grill marks, if desired.) Transfer the steak to a cutting board and let rest for 5 to 8 minutes.

6. Thinly slice the steak across the grain. Transfer to a platter and serve with the chimichurri sauce and lime wedges.

P/E ratio **2.1** • calories **202** • fat **10g** • protein **25g** • carbs **3g** • fiber **1g**

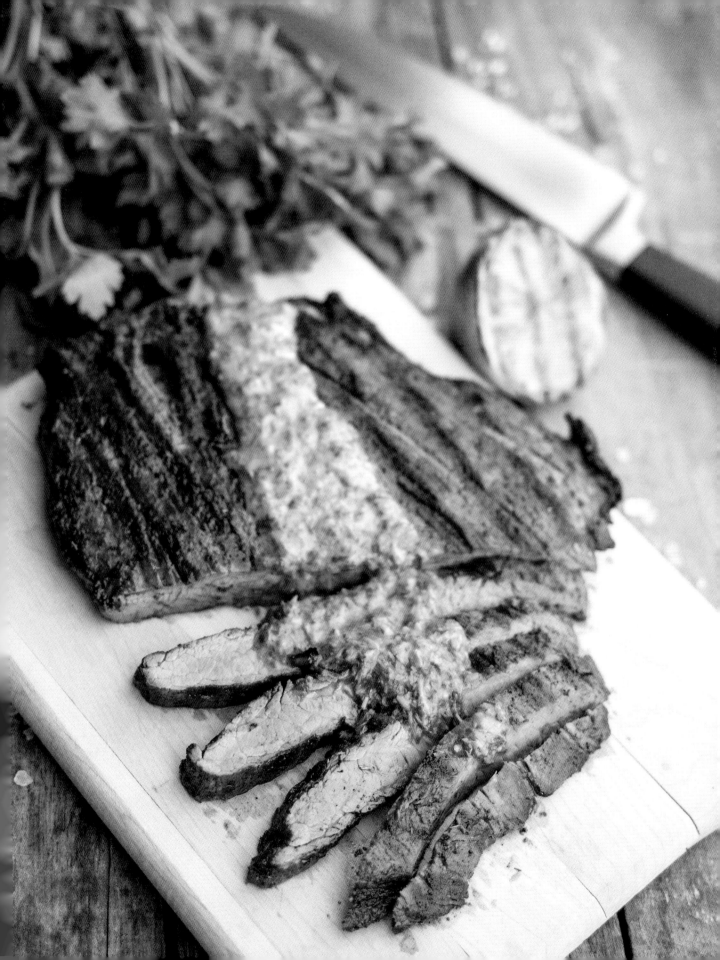

BBQ Meatloaf

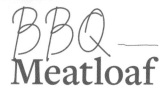

  yield: 6 servings • prep time: 10 minutes, plus 15 minutes to rest (not including time to make sauce) • cook time: 45 minutes

2 pounds 95% lean ground beef

1 cup finely diced button mushrooms

¼ cup finely diced yellow onions

2 tablespoons prepared yellow mustard

1 large egg white

1 tablespoon fine sea salt

½ teaspoon freshly ground black pepper

1 teaspoon liquid smoke (optional)

¾ cup BBQ Sauce (page 102), divided

1. Preheat the oven to 350°F. Line a 9 by 5-inch loaf pan with parchment paper.

2. Put the ground beef, mushrooms, onions, mustard, egg white, salt, pepper, and liquid smoke, if using, in a large bowl. Using your hands, mix the ingredients until well combined. Press the mixture into the prepared pan.

3. Bake the meatloaf until the internal temperature reaches 160°F, 45 to 55 minutes.

4. Remove the pan from the oven, spread ½ cup of the BBQ sauce on top of the meatloaf, and bake for 5 more minutes. Let the meatloaf rest for 15 minutes.

5. Cut the meatloaf into 6 slices and serve with the remaining ¼ cup of BBQ sauce.

P/E ratio 3.7 • calories 280 • fat 10g • protein 43g • carbs 2g • fiber 0.4g

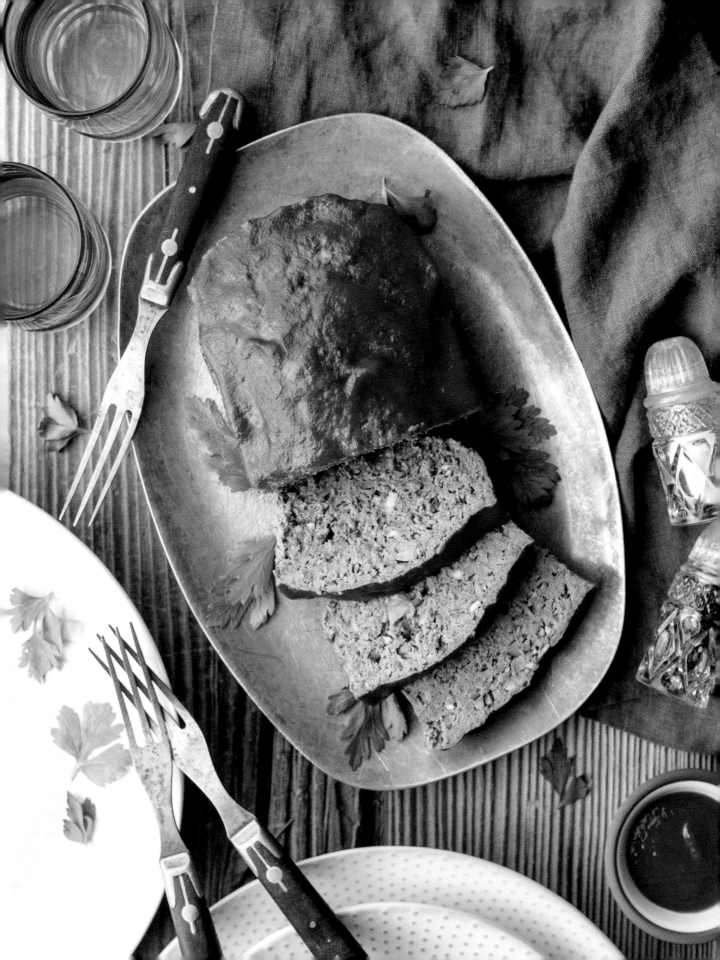

Asian-Style Meatballs

  yield: 6 servings • prep time: 8 minutes • cook time: 15 minutes

2 pounds 95% lean ground beef

2 large egg whites

¾ cup finely chopped button mushrooms

¼ cup thinly sliced green onions

2 teaspoons peeled and grated fresh ginger

1 clove garlic, minced

1½ teaspoons wheat-free tamari

1 teaspoon red pepper flakes

⅛ teaspoon liquid stevia

Fried "Rice" (page 226), for serving (optional)

1. Preheat the oven to 400°F. Line a rimmed baking sheet with parchment paper.

2. Place the ground beef, egg whites, mushrooms, green onions, ginger, garlic, tamari, red pepper flakes, and stevia in a large bowl. Using your hands, mix the ingredients until well combined. Shape the mixture into 1¼-inch balls and arrange on the prepared baking sheet.

3. Bake the meatballs until golden brown on the outside and no longer pink inside, about 15 minutes.

4. Serve the meatballs over fried "rice," if desired.

P/E ratio **4.0** • calories **316** • fat **10g** • protein **51g** • carbs **3g** • fiber **0.4g**

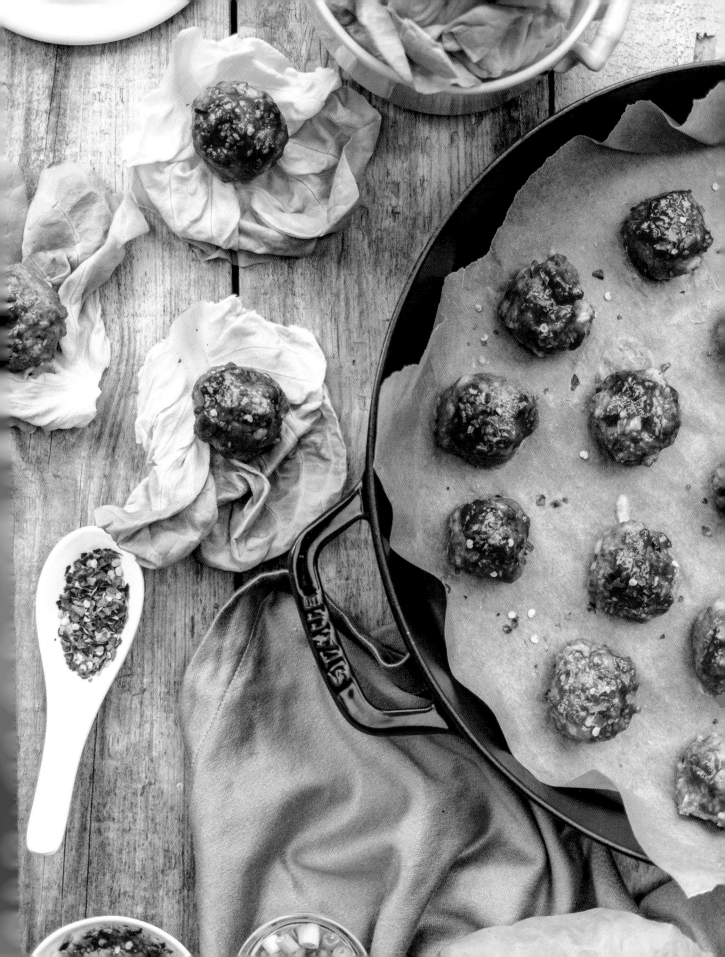

Sweet and Sour Pork Chops

   yield: 4 servings • prep time: 5 minutes • cook time: 16 minutes

1 teaspoon coconut oil, lard, or tallow

4 (5-ounce) bone-in pork chops, visible fat removed

1 teaspoon fine sea salt

½ teaspoon freshly ground black pepper

Sweet and Sour Sauce:

½ cup chicken broth

⅓ cup confectioners'-style erythritol or equivalent amount of powdered or liquid sweetener

⅓ cup wheat-free tamari

¼ cup tomato sauce

1 tablespoon coconut vinegar or apple cider vinegar

1 clove garlic, minced

¼ teaspoon peeled and grated fresh ginger

Green onions, sliced on the diagonal, for garnish (optional)

1. Heat the oil in a large cast-iron skillet over medium-high heat.

2. Pat the pork chops dry with paper towels and sprinkle both sides with the salt and pepper.

3. When the oil is hot, cook the chops until golden brown on one side, about 3 minutes. Flip them over and cook until the other side is golden brown and the internal temperature reaches 145°F, about 3 minutes more. (Do not overcrowd the pan; if necessary, cook the chops in batches.) Remove the chops from the skillet and set aside to rest, keeping the pan on the heat; leave the drippings in the pan.

4. While the chops rest, make the sauce: Add the broth, sweetener, tamari, tomato sauce, vinegar, garlic, and ginger to the drippings in the skillet and whisk to combine. Simmer until the sauce is reduced a bit and thickened, about 10 minutes.

5. Serve the chops with the sauce. Garnish with green onions, if desired.

P/E ratio **2.3** • calories **406** • fat **18g** • protein **54g** • carbs **6g** • fiber **0.4g**

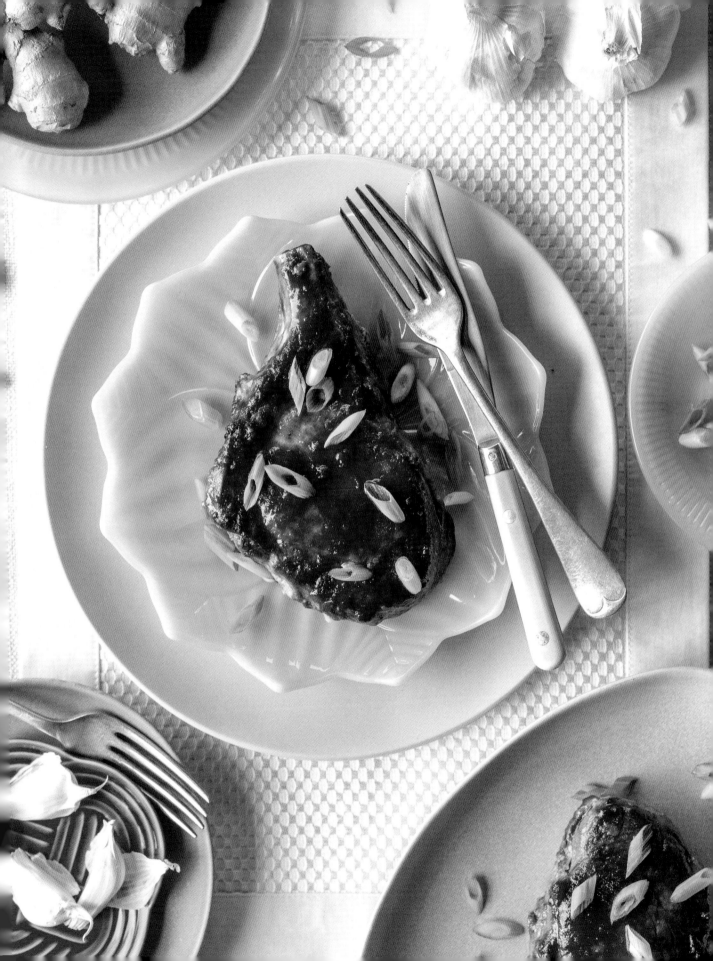

Garlic-Thyme
Pork Tenderloins

   yield: 12 servings • prep time: 5 minutes, plus 10 minutes to rest • cook time: 40 minutes

2 (2-pound) pork tenderloins

8 cloves garlic, halved lengthwise

1 tablespoon fresh thyme leaves, finely chopped

1½ teaspoons fine sea salt

1 teaspoon freshly ground black pepper

¼ cup apple cider vinegar

1. Preheat the oven to 350°F. Line a 9 by 13-inch baking dish with parchment paper.

2. Place the pork tenderloins in the prepared baking dish. Using the tip of a paring knife, make 8 pockets all over each tenderloin. Tuck a garlic clove half into each pocket. Season the tenderloins on all sides with the thyme, salt, and pepper. Pour the vinegar into the baking dish.

3. Bake until the internal temperature of the pork reaches 145°F, about 40 minutes. Transfer the pork to a cutting board to rest for 10 minutes.

4. Cut the pork into ½-inch slices and arrange on a platter. Spoon the juices from the baking dish over them before serving.

P/E ratio **3.5** • calories **423** • fat **16g** • protein **62g** • carbs **2g** • fiber **0.3g**

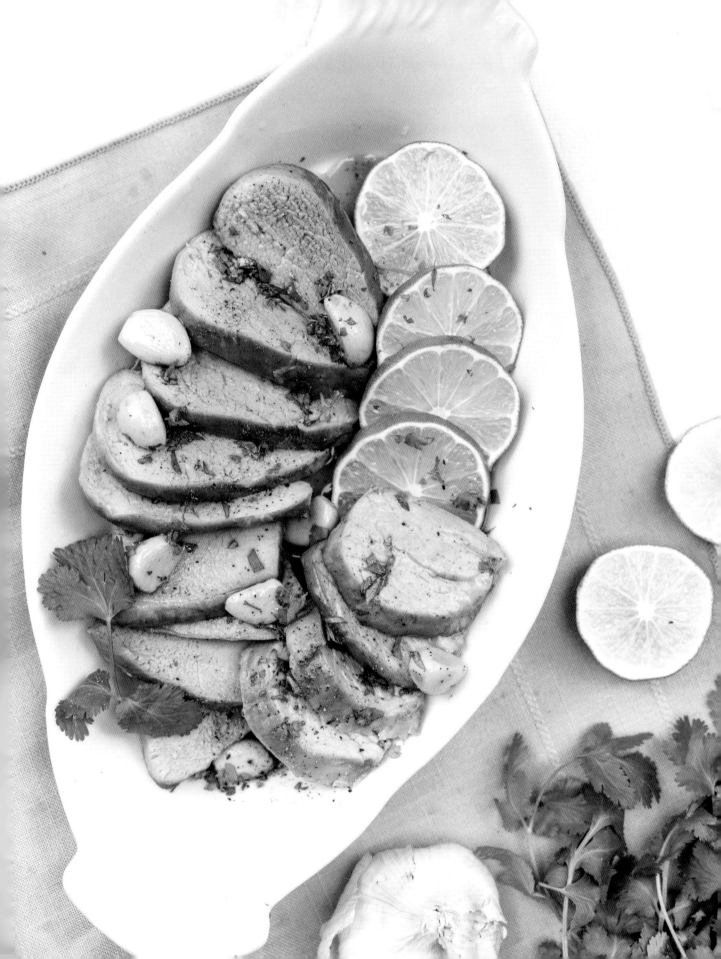

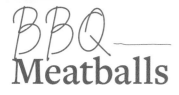

BBQ Meatballs

  yield: 8 servings • prep time: 10 minutes • cook time: 15 minutes

2 pounds 95% lean ground beef

¼ cup chopped yellow onions

1 clove garlic, minced

1 tablespoon prepared yellow mustard

2 teaspoons fine sea salt

1 teaspoon dried thyme leaves

1 egg white

BBQ Sauce:

¼ cup chicken or beef broth

¼ cup tomato sauce

2 tablespoons apple cider vinegar

1 teaspoon garlic powder

1 teaspoon onion powder

¼ teaspoon fine sea salt

⅛ teaspoon liquid smoke (optional)

⅛ teaspoon liquid stevia, or more to taste

Chopped fresh parsley leaves, for garnish (optional)

1. Preheat the oven to 425°F. Line a rimmed baking sheet with parchment paper.

2. Make the meatballs: Put the ground beef, onions, garlic, mustard, salt, thyme, and egg white in a large bowl. Using your hands, mix the ingredients until well combined. Shape the mixture into 1¼-inch balls and arrange on the prepared baking sheet.

3. Bake the meatballs until cooked through and no longer pink inside, about 15 minutes.

4. Meanwhile, make the sauce: Put all of the ingredients in a small saucepan. Simmer over medium-high heat until the sauce has reduced a bit and thickened, about 10 minutes. Taste and adjust the seasoning and sweetness to your liking.

5. Serve the meatballs with the sauce. Garnish with parsley, if desired.

P/E ratio **4.1** • calories **208** • fat **7g** • protein **32g** • carbs **1g** • fiber **0.2g**

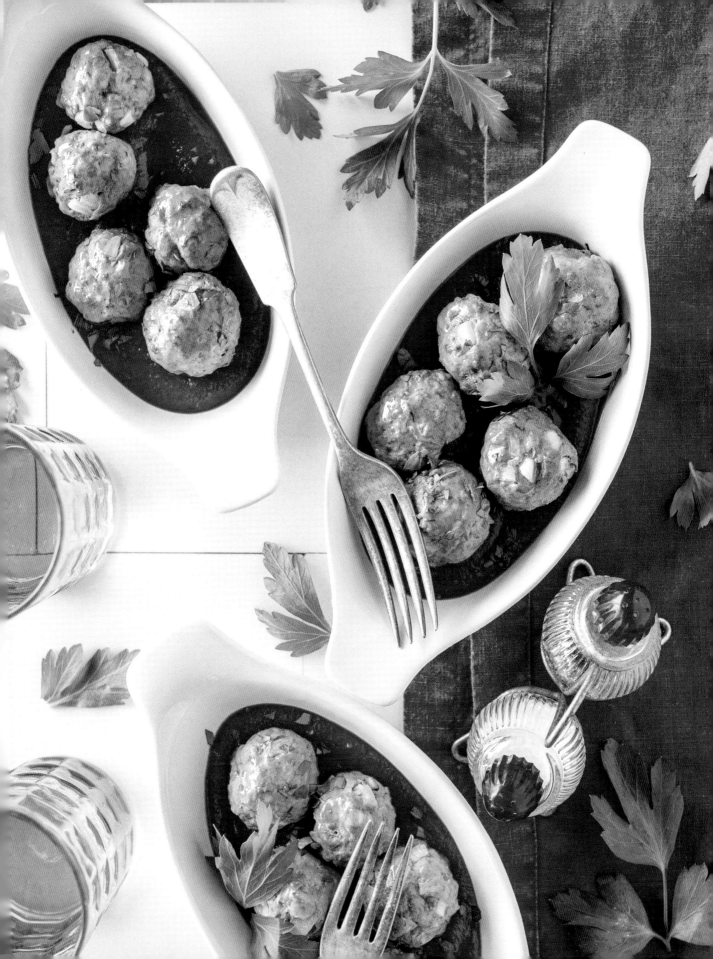

Grilled Pork Chops
with Truffle Mustard Sauce

   yield: 2 servings • prep time: 5 minutes, plus 10 minutes to rest (not including time to make sauce) • cook time: 6 minutes

Duck fat or coconut oil, for greasing

4 (5-ounce) boneless pork chops, visible fat removed

1 teaspoon fine sea salt

½ teaspoon freshly ground black pepper

¼ cup Truffle Mustard Sauce (page 100), for serving

1. Lightly grease the grates of a grill with duck fat. Heat the grill to medium-high heat.

2. Pat the pork chops dry with paper towels and season on both sides with the salt and pepper.

3. Grill the pork chops until golden brown on one side, about 3 minutes; flip and grill until the other side is golden brown and the internal temperature reaches 145°F, about 3 minutes more. Remove the chops from the grill and set aside to rest for 10 minutes.

4. Cut the chops into slices and sprinkle with more pepper. Serve with the truffle mustard sauce.

P/E ratio **2.6** • calories **317** • fat **15g** • protein **42g** • carbs **1g** • fiber **0.1g**

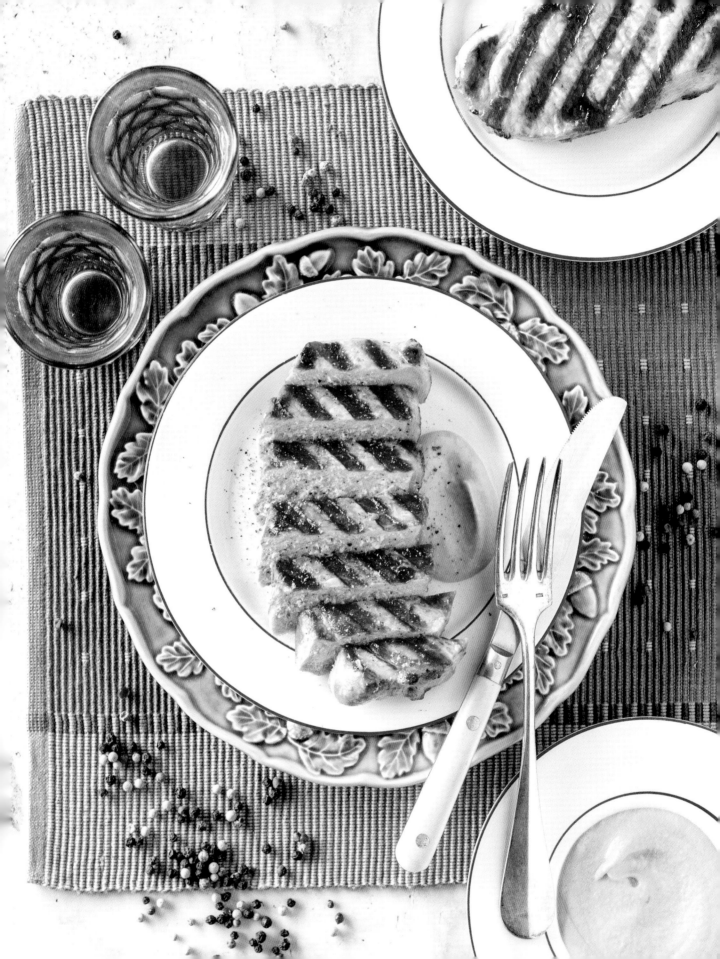

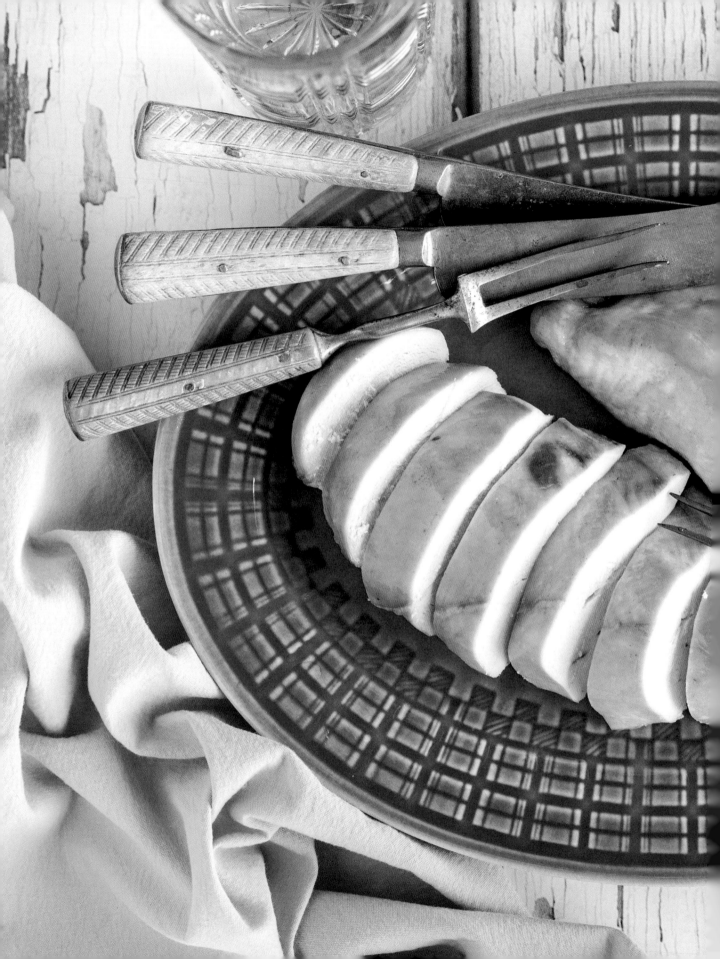

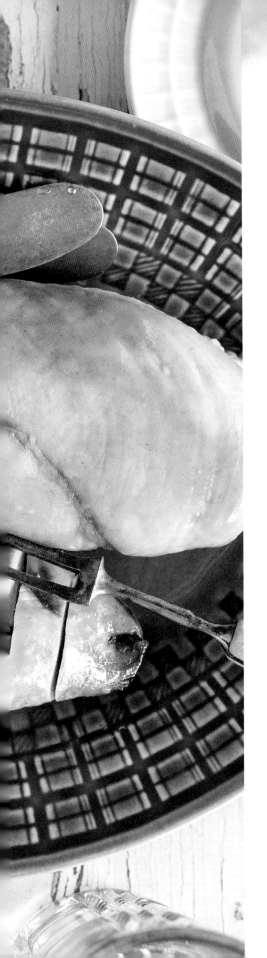

Slow Cooker Ranch Chicken / 120

BBQ Chicken Flatbread / 122

Smoked Chicken Breasts / 124

Chicken Strips with Carolina BBQ Sauce / 126

Grilled Chicken Breasts with
Carolina BBQ Sauce / 128

Poached Chicken Breasts / 129

Egg Foo Young / 130

Mojito Chicken / 132

BBQ Grilled Chicken / 134

Asian-Inspired Stir-Fried Turkey / 136

Grilled Chicken Breasts with
Tomato Basil Sauce / 138

Saltimbocca-Style Chicken Breasts / 140

Orange Chicken / 142

Chicken Fried "Rice" / 144

Thanksgiving Turkey Breast / 146

Bourbon Chicken / 148

Buffalo Chicken Meatballs / 150

Baked Chicken Breasts with Ginger Sauce / 152

Turkey Meatloaf with Dijon Sauce / 154

Slow Cooker Doro Wat / 156

Slow Cooker Ranch Chicken

    yield: 4 servings • prep time: 5 minutes • cook time: 4 to 8 hours

4 (6-ounce) boneless, skinless chicken breasts

1 cup chicken broth

2 tablespoons dried parsley

1 tablespoon onion powder

2 teaspoons garlic powder

1½ teaspoons dried dill weed

1 teaspoon dried chives

1 teaspoon fine sea salt

1 teaspoon freshly ground black pepper

Chopped fresh parsley leaves, for garnish (optional)

1. Place all of the ingredients in a 4-quart slow cooker. Cover and cook on low for 6 to 8 hours or on high for 4 hours, until tender.

2. Shred the chicken with two forks and mix it well with the sauce.

3. Garnish with parsley, if desired, and serve.

P/E ratio **3.3** • calories **361** • fat **15g** • protein **52g** • carbs **2g** • fiber **1g**

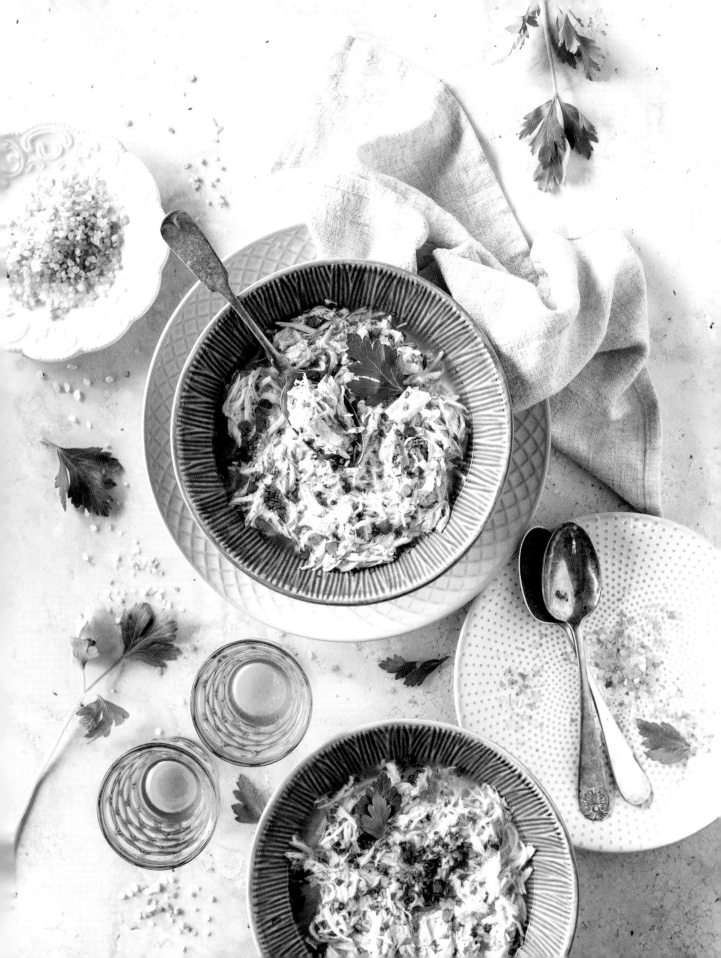

BBQ
Chicken Flatbread

  yield: 4 servings • prep time: 15 minutes (not including time to make sauce or chicken) • cook time: 15 minutes

Crust:

6 large egg whites

½ cup unflavored egg white protein powder

2 teaspoons smoked paprika (optional)

1 cup BBQ Sauce (page 102)

2 pieces BBQ Grilled Chicken (page 134), cut into ¼-inch dice

¼ cup red onion slices

Chopped fresh parsley leaves, for garnish

1. Preheat the oven to 350°F. Line a baking sheet with parchment paper.

2. Make the crust: Put the egg whites in a large bowl and beat with an electric hand mixer on high speed until stiff peaks form, about 10 minutes. Add the protein powder and paprika, if using, and beat on low, being careful not to deflate the whites.

3. Use a rubber spatula to spread the crust mixture on the prepared baking sheet, forming a 12-inch circle. Smooth out the top and bake until golden brown, 10 to 15 minutes.

4. Remove the baking sheet from the oven and spread the BBQ sauce on the crust. Top with the diced chicken. Return the baking sheet to the oven and bake until the chicken is warmed through, about 5 minutes.

5. Arrange the red onion slices on top and garnish with parsley. Cut into slices and serve.

P/E ratio **4.1** • calories **256** • fat **7g** • protein **41g** • carbs **5g** • fiber **2g**

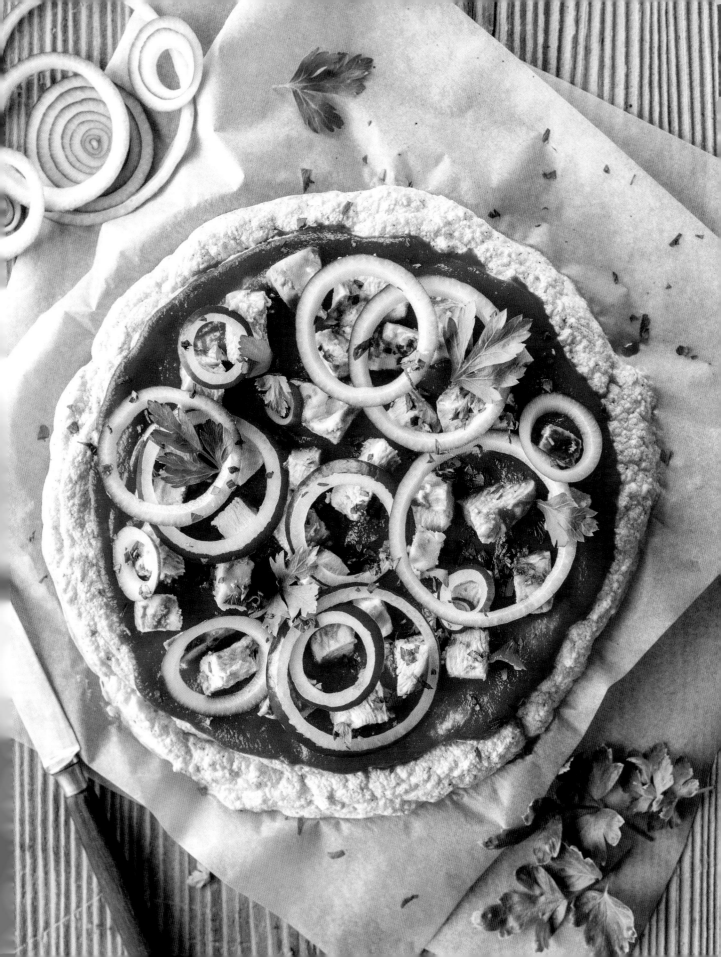

Smoked Chicken Breasts

   yield: 8 servings • prep time: 5 minutes, plus 30 minutes to soak wood chips (not including time to make sauce) • cook time: 1 hour 15 minutes

Smoking foods sounds intimidating, but it is really quite simple! It's important that you read the manufacturer's directions for your smoker before you begin. There are several types of smokers—wood, electric, propane, and more—and each type works differently. A thermometer to monitor the temperature of the smoker is also essential when it comes to slow-cooking meat.

4 pounds boneless, skinless chicken breasts

1 teaspoon fine sea salt

½ teaspoon freshly ground black pepper

1 cup BBQ Sauce (page 102), for serving

Special Equipment:

Smoker

1. About 30 minutes before you're ready to smoke the chicken, remove the chicken from the refrigerator. Pat it dry with paper towels and season it on all sides with the salt and pepper.

2. Set the smoker temperature to 180°F.

3. Smoke the chicken for 30 minutes. Increase the heat to 230°F and continue cooking until the internal temperature of the chicken reaches 162°F, 45 minutes to 1 hour. Remove the chicken from the smoker and let it rest until the internal temperature rises to 165°F, 5 to 10 minutes.

4. Slice the chicken and serve it with the BBQ sauce.

P/E ratio **3.9** • calories **444** • fat **17g** • protein **67g** • carbs **0.1g** • fiber **0g**

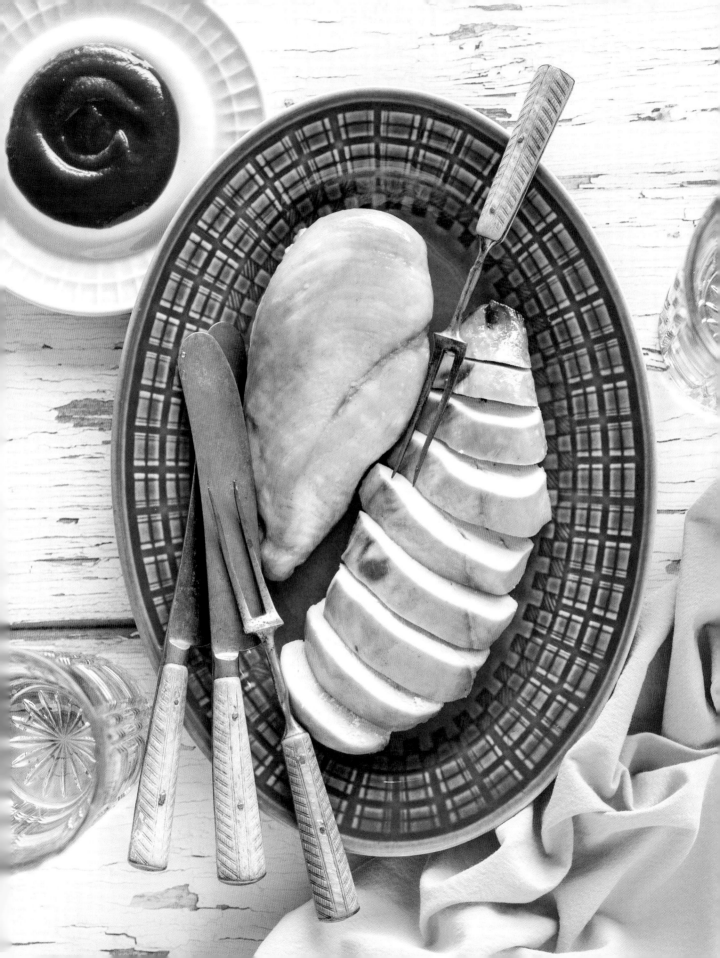

Chicken Strips
with Carolina BBQ Sauce

   yield: 8 servings • prep time: 5 minutes (not including time to make sauce) • cook time: 15 minutes

1 lemon, thinly sliced

4 (6-ounce) boneless, skinless chicken breasts, cut into 1-inch-wide strips

2 tablespoons lemon pepper seasoning

½ cup Carolina BBQ Sauce (page 267)

1. Preheat the oven to 400°F.

2. Arrange the lemon slices on a rimmed baking sheet or in a 9 by 13-inch baking dish.

3. Pat the chicken strips dry with paper towels. Coat the chicken thoroughly with the lemon pepper seasoning. Arrange the strips on top of the lemon slices. Bake until the chicken is no longer pink inside, 18 to 20 minutes.

4. Serve the chicken with the BBQ sauce.

P/E ratio **3.4** • calories **465** • fat **19g** • protein **67g** • carbs **2g** • fiber **1g**

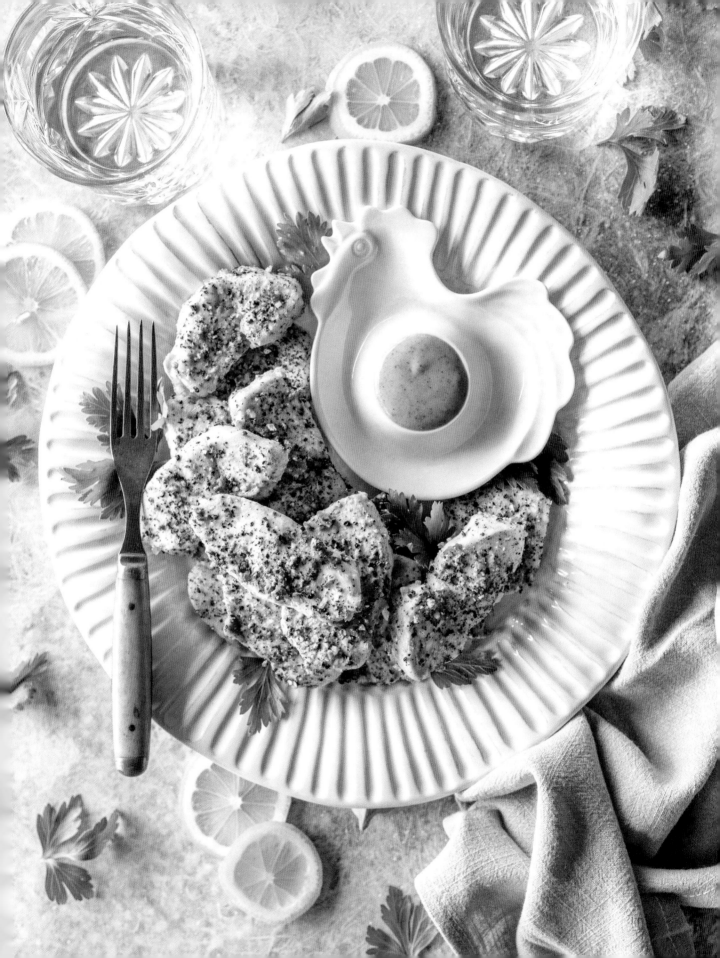

Grilled Chicken Breasts
with Carolina BBQ Sauce

   yield: 4 servings • prep time: 7 minutes, plus 5 minutes to rest (not including time to make sauce) • cook time: 15 minutes

Duck fat or coconut oil, for greasing

4 (6-ounce) boneless skinless chicken breasts

2 teaspoons fine sea salt

2 teaspoons freshly ground black pepper

½ teaspoon garlic powder

½ cup Carolina BBQ Sauce (page 267)

Fresh parsley leaves, for garnish

1. Lightly grease the grates of a grill with duck fat. Heat the grill to medium-high heat.

2. Pat the chicken dry with paper towels. Season on both sides with the salt, pepper, and garlic powder. When the grill is hot, grill the chicken, covered, for 8 minutes. Turn the heat down to low, flip the chicken, and continue to grill until the internal temperature reaches 162°F, about 8 minutes more. Transfer the chicken to a serving platter and let it rest until the internal temperature reaches 165°F, 5 to 10 minutes.

3. Drizzle the chicken with the BBQ sauce, garnish with parsley, and serve.

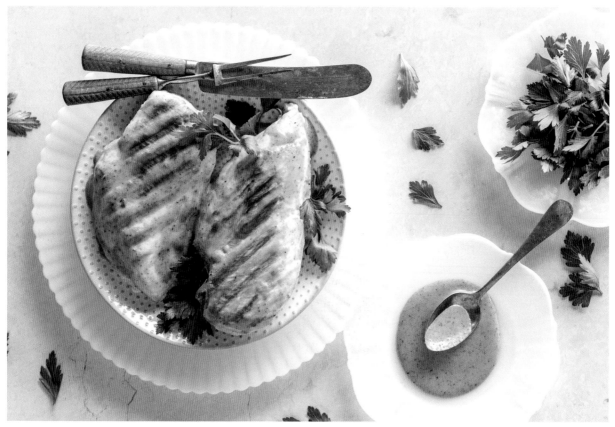

P/E ratio **3.1** • calories **334** • fat **14g** • protein **47g** • carbs **2g** • fiber **1g**

Poached
Chicken Breasts

   yield: 4 servings • prep time: 5 minutes • cook time: 20 minutes

4 (6-ounce) boneless, skinless chicken breasts

1 shallot, peeled and quartered

3 cloves garlic, minced

3 sprigs fresh thyme, or 1 teaspoon dried thyme leaves

2 bay leaves

1½ teaspoons fine sea salt

5 cups chicken broth or water

1. Put the chicken, shallot, garlic, thyme, bay leaves, and salt in a medium-sized saucepan. Cover with the broth and bring to a low simmer over high heat. (This will take a few minutes. For the most tender poached chicken, do not rush this step.)

2. Reduce the heat to low and cook until the internal temperature of the chicken reaches 162°F, 10 to 15 minutes. Remove the pan from the heat and allow the chicken to rest until the internal temperature reaches 165°F, 5 to 10 minutes.

3. Cut the chicken into thick slices and serve.

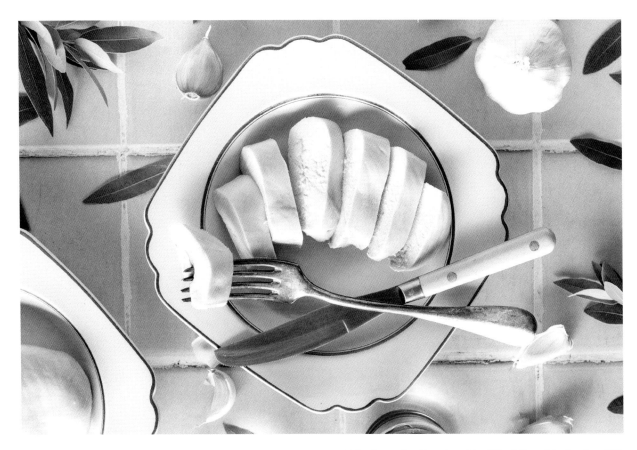

P/E ratio 7.0 • calories 238 • fat 5g • protein 48g • carbs 2g • fiber 0.1g   The Protein-Sparing Modified Fast Method

Egg Foo Young

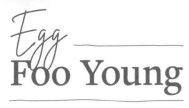

yield: 8 omelets (2 per serving) • prep time: 10 minutes • cook time: 15 minutes

Egg foo young can be served as a main dish over "Fried" Rice (page 226), and it also makes for a filling snack.

Sauce:

¾ cup chicken broth

¼ cup wheat-free tamari

½ teaspoon hot sauce

1 teaspoon peeled and grated fresh ginger, divided

⅛ teaspoon liquid stevia (optional)

½ teaspoon grass-fed powdered gelatin

Omelets:

12 large egg whites, or 1½ cups 100% liquid egg whites

6 ounces deli turkey or chicken, finely chopped

2 ounces button mushrooms, stemmed and thinly sliced

½ cup thinly sliced green onions, plus more for garnish

¼ cup thinly sliced green or napa cabbage

2 teaspoons peeled and grated fresh ginger

1 large clove garlic, minced

½ teaspoon fine sea salt

½ teaspoon freshly ground black pepper

Duck fat spray or coconut oil spray, for greasing

1. Make the sauce: Combine the broth, tamari, hot sauce, ginger, and stevia, if using, in a small saucepan. Whisk in the gelatin. Bring to a boil over medium-high heat and cook, uncovered, until the sauce has reduced to about ½ cup, 5 to 10 minutes. Keep warm.

2. Make the omelets: In a large bowl, whisk the egg whites just until well blended. Stir in the turkey, mushrooms, green onions, cabbage, ginger, garlic, salt, and pepper.

3. Lightly grease a large skillet with duck fat spray and place it over medium heat. When hot, pour in ½ cup of the egg white mixture to make an omelet. Cook 4 omelets at a time until golden on both sides, 2 to 3 minutes per side. Transfer the omelets to a serving platter. Spray the skillet with duck fat spray and repeat with the remaining egg white mixture, making 4 more omelets.

4. Put 2 omelets on each plate and top with 2 tablespoons of the sauce. Garnish with more green onions and serve warm.

P/E ratio **4.0** • calories **164** • fat **4g** • protein **28g** • carbs **4g** • fiber **1g**

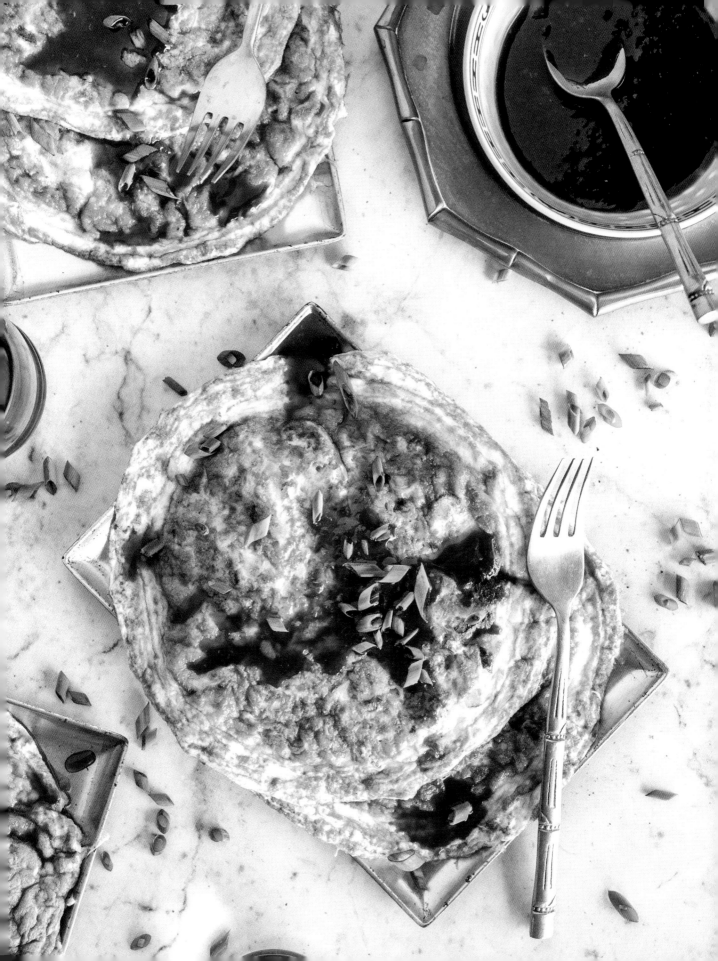

Mojito Chicken

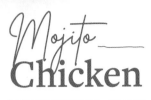

   yield: 6 servings • prep time: 7 minutes, plus 3 hours to marinate • cook time: 30 minutes

¾ cup fresh lime juice

¼ cup avocado oil

½ cup finely chopped fresh mint

2 teaspoons minced garlic

1 tablespoon fine sea salt

6 (6-ounce) boneless, skinless chicken breasts

Fresh mint leaves, thinly sliced, for garnish

2 small limes, sliced, for serving

1. Place the lime juice, oil, mint, garlic, and salt in a large shallow baking dish. Add the chicken and roll around to coat well. Cover and refrigerate for at least 3 hours or overnight.

2. Lightly grease the grates of a grill with duck fat. Heat the grill to medium-high heat.

3. When the grill is hot, remove the chicken from the marinade and discard the marinade. Grill the chicken, covered, for 8 minutes. Turn the heat down to low, flip the chicken, and continue to grill until the internal temperature reaches 162°F, about 8 minutes longer. Transfer the chicken to a serving platter and let rest until the internal temperature reaches 165°F, 5 to 10 minutes.

4. Cut the chicken into thick slices. Garnish with mint and serve with lime slices.

P/E ratio **1.6** • calories **282** • fat **17g** • protein **29g** • carbs **1g** • fiber **0.1g**

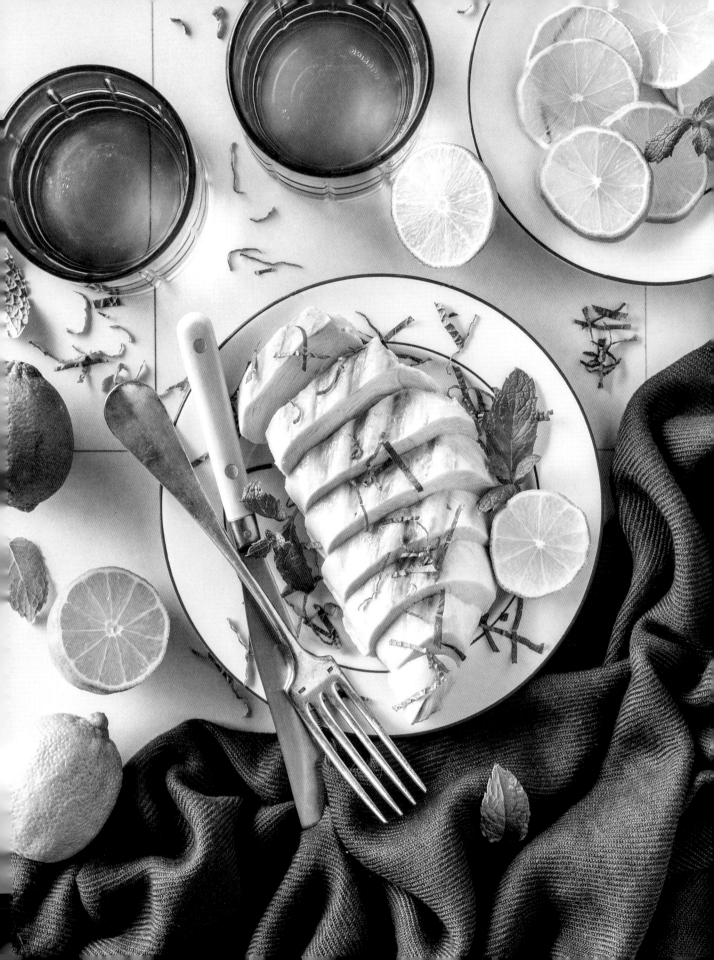

BBQ
Grilled Chicken

   yield: 6 servings • prep time: 7 minutes (not including time to make sauce) • cook time: 30 minutes

Duck fat or coconut oil, for greasing

6 (6-ounce) boneless, skinless chicken breasts

1½ teaspoons fine sea salt

1 teaspoon smoked paprika

¾ cup BBQ Sauce (page 102), divided

1. Lightly grease the grates of a grill with duck fat. Heat the grill to medium-high heat.

2. Pat the chicken breasts dry with paper towels. Season on all sides with the salt and paprika.

3. When the grill is hot, grill the chicken, covered, for 8 minutes. Turn the heat down to low, flip the chicken, and continue to grill until the internal temperature registers 162°F, about 8 minutes more.

4. Brush the chicken with ¼ cup of the BBQ sauce and grill for another 30 seconds. Transfer to a serving platter and let rest until the internal temperature reaches 165°F, 5 to 10 minutes.

5. Garnish with parsley, if desired, and serve the chicken with the remaining ½ cup of BBQ sauce.

P/E ratio **1.8** • calories **534** • fat **30g** • protein **59g** • carbs **3g** • fiber **1g**

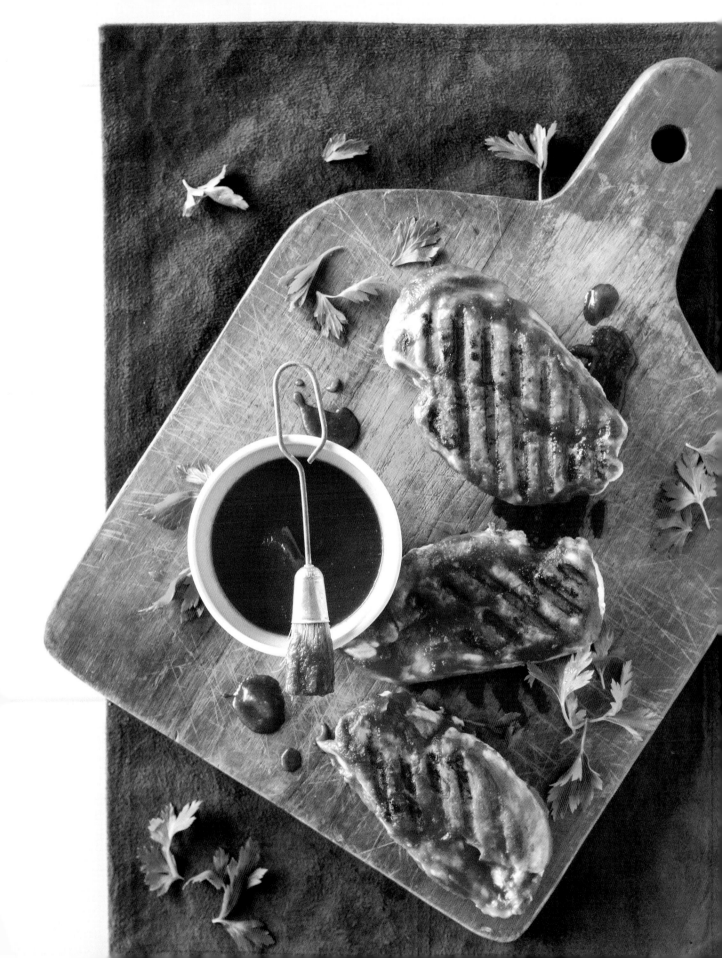

Asian-Inspired
Stir-Fried Turkey

   yield: 3 servings • prep time: 5 minutes • cook time: 6 minutes

1½ teaspoons toasted sesame oil

3 cloves garlic, minced

1 green onion, sliced, plus more for garnish if desired

1 pound 95% lean ground turkey or ground chicken

2 tablespoons wheat-free tamari

1 teaspoon peeled and grated fresh ginger

1 teaspoon distilled white vinegar

¼ teaspoon fine sea salt

½ teaspoon freshly ground black pepper

¼ teaspoon liquid stevia

Red pepper flakes, to taste (optional)

1. Heat the oil in a large skillet over medium heat. Add the garlic and green onion; sauté for 1 minute.

2. Add the ground turkey, tamari, ginger, vinegar, salt, pepper, stevia, and red pepper flakes, if using. Cook, breaking up the turkey into small pieces with a spatula, until no pink remains, about 5 minutes.

3. Garnish with extra green onions, if desired. Serve warm.

P/E ratio **1.7** • calories **400** • fat **23g** • protein **43g** • carbs **3g** • fiber **0.5g**

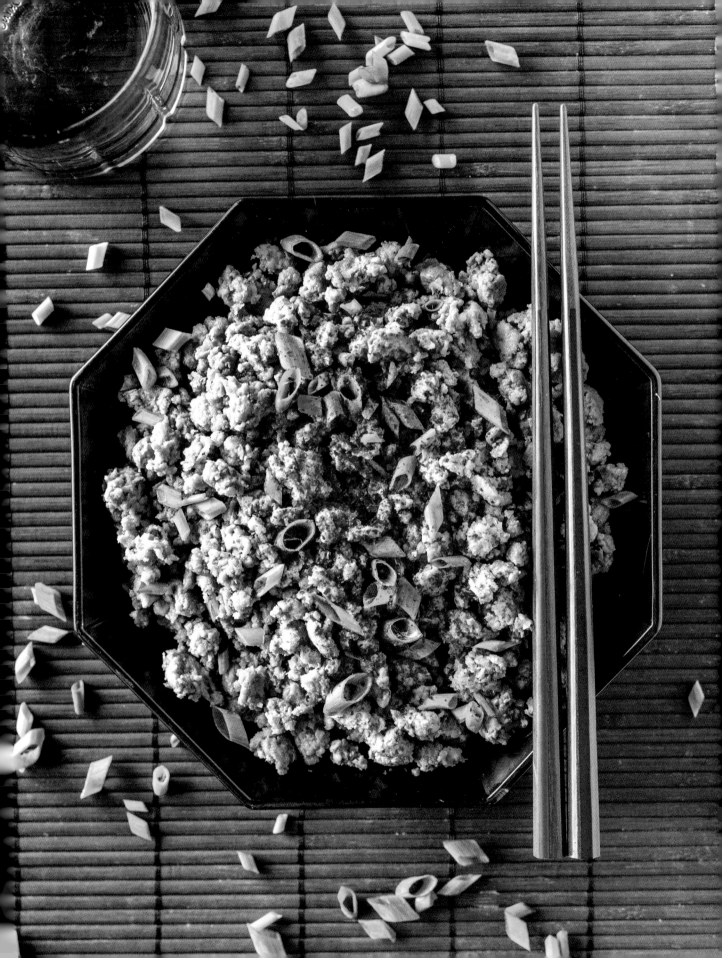

Grilled Chicken Breasts
with Tomato Basil Sauce

   yield: 4 servings • prep time: 8 minutes • cook time: 25 minutes

This tomato basil sauce is on the thin side—almost brothlike—but it is very flavorful!

Duck fat or coconut oil, for greasing

4 (6-ounce) boneless, skinless chicken breasts

2 tablespoons dried basil leaves

1 teaspoon garlic powder

1 teaspoon fine sea salt

1 teaspoon freshly ground black pepper

Sauce:

2 cups beef broth

½ cup tomato sauce

2 tablespoons chopped fresh basil leaves, or 2 teaspoons dried basil leaves

2 cloves garlic, minced

¼ teaspoon fine sea salt

⅛ teaspoon liquid stevia (optional)

1. Lightly grease the grates of a grill with duck fat. Heat the grill to medium-high heat.

2. Pat the chicken breasts dry with paper towels and season on both sides with the dried basil, garlic powder, salt, and pepper.

3. When the grill is hot, grill the chicken, covered, for 8 minutes. Turn the heat down to low, flip the chicken, and continue to grill until the internal temperature reaches 162°F, about 8 minutes more. Remove the chicken from the grill and let it rest until the internal temperature reaches 165°F, 5 to 10 minutes.

4. Make the sauce: Combine the broth, tomato sauce, basil, garlic, and salt in a medium-sized saucepan and bring to a boil over high heat. Continue to boil over high heat, uncovered, until the sauce has reduced slightly and thickened up a bit (it will still be quite thin), about 10 minutes. Taste and add the stevia, if using.

5. Serve the chicken with the sauce.

P/E ratio **5.3** • calories **193** • fat **4g** • protein **37g** • carbs **4g** • fiber **1g**

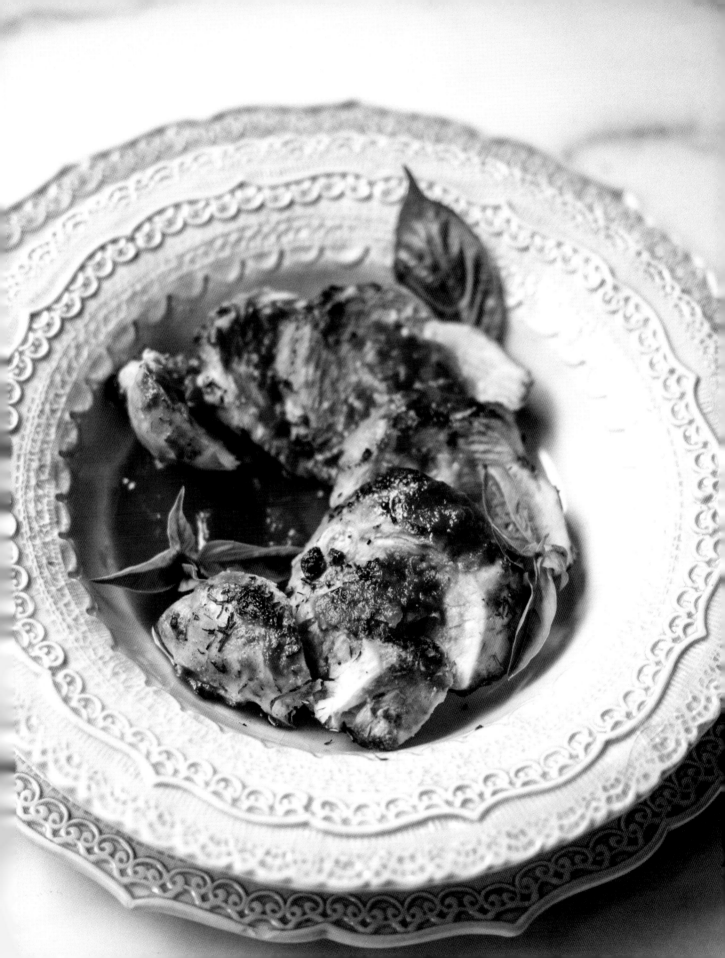

Saltimbocca-Style Chicken Breasts

   yield: 4 servings • prep time: 10 minutes • cook time: 20 minutes

4 (6-ounce) boneless, skinless chicken breasts

½ cup finely chopped fresh parsley leaves

¼ cup finely chopped fresh chives

4 cloves garlic, peeled

2 tablespoons lemon juice

1 teaspoon ground fennel

1 teaspoon finely chopped fresh rosemary

1 teaspoon dried rubbed sage

½ teaspoon red pepper flakes

3 teaspoons fine sea salt

4 thin slices 95% lean ham

1. Preheat the oven to 350°F. Line a rimmed baking sheet with parchment paper.

2. Using a meat mallet, pound the chicken breasts evenly on both sides until they are ¼ inch thick.

3. Put the parsley, chives, garlic cloves, lemon juice, fennel, rosemary, sage, red pepper flakes, and salt in a food processor; blend into a smooth paste.

4. Rub one-quarter of the paste on one side of each chicken breast and lay a slice of ham on top. Roll the chicken breasts up tightly like a jelly roll; secure with toothpicks.

5. Arrange the chicken rolls on the prepared baking sheet and bake until the internal temperature reaches 162°F, about 20 minutes. Let rest until the internal temperature reaches 165°F, 5 to 10 minutes.

6. Cut the chicken rolls into thick slices and serve warm.

P/E ratio **4.9** • calories **214** • fat **6g** • protein **39g** • carbs **3g** • fiber **1g**

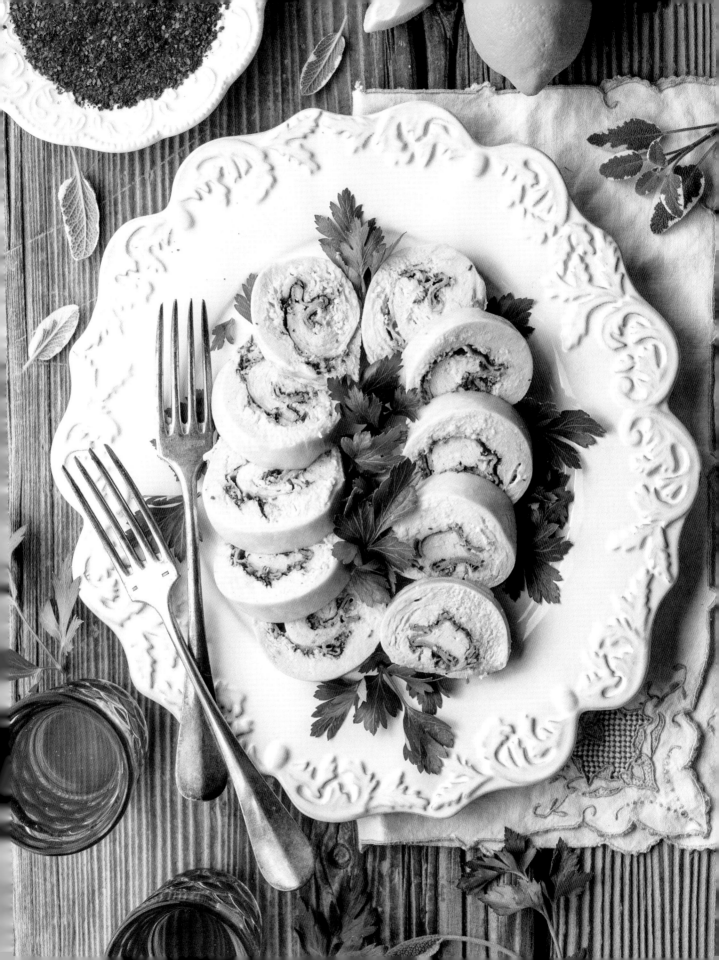

Orange Chicken

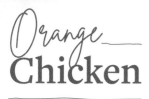

   yield: 4 servings • prep time: 5 minutes (not including time to make marmalade) • cook time: 20 minutes

1 teaspoon coconut oil, lard, or tallow

2 pounds boneless, skinless chicken breasts, cut into bite-sized pieces

½ teaspoon fine sea salt

¾ cup Orange Marmalade (page 262)

⅓ cup wheat-free tamari

1 tablespoon coconut vinegar or apple cider vinegar

1 clove garlic, minced

¼ teaspoon peeled and grated fresh ginger

Green onions, sliced on the diagonal, for garnish (optional)

Fried "Rice" (page 226), for serving (optional)

1. Heat the oil in a wok or large cast-iron skillet over medium-high heat. When the wok is hot, add the chicken and stir-fry on all sides until light golden brown, about 4 minutes. Remove the chicken from the wok and set aside.

2. Add the marmalade, tamari, vinegar, garlic, and ginger to the wok and stir to combine. Simmer until the sauce thickens to the consistency of loose jelly, about 10 minutes.

3. Return the chicken to the wok and simmer until the sauce forms a thick glaze coating the chicken, 5 to 10 minutes.

4. Garnish with green onions, if using, and serve over fried "rice," if desired.

P/E ratio 5.7 • calories 308 • fat 7g • protein 61g • carbs 4g • fiber 0.3g

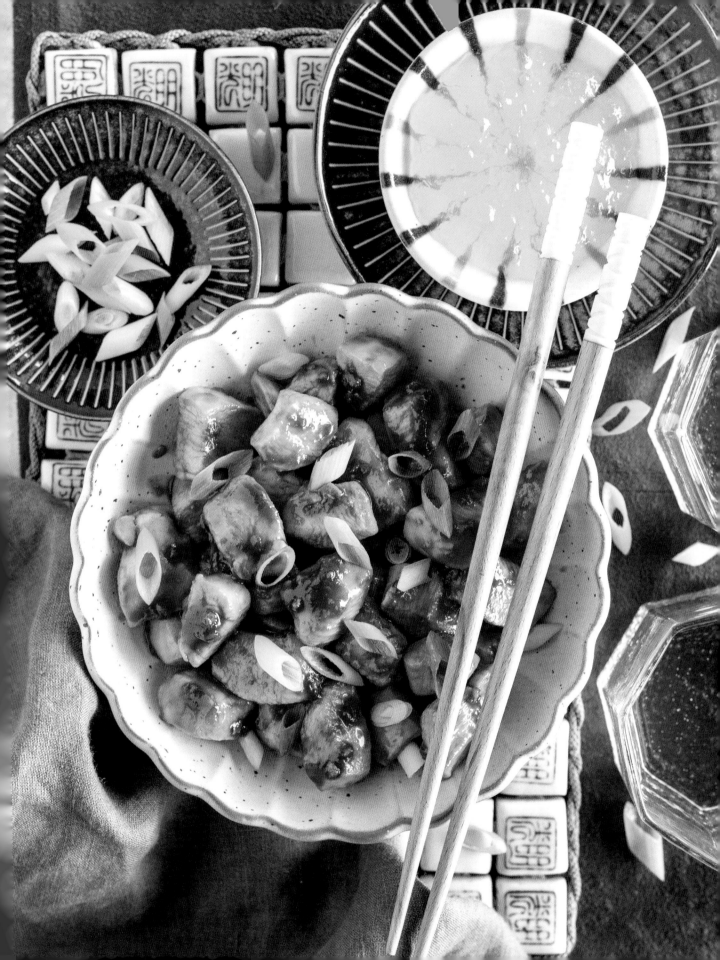

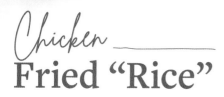

Chicken
Fried "Rice"

  yield: 4 servings • prep time: 5 minutes • cook time: 11 minutes

12 large egg whites

½ cup beef broth

2 teaspoons wheat-free tamari

1 teaspoon fine sea salt

½ teaspoon freshly ground black pepper

1 teaspoon coconut oil, lard, or tallow

¼ cup diced yellow onions

1 clove garlic, minced

1 pound extra-lean ground chicken or 95% lean ground turkey

For Garnish (optional):

1 teaspoon red pepper flakes

Thinly sliced green onions

1. In a large bowl, whisk the egg whites, broth, tamari, salt, and pepper until well combined.

2. Heat the oil in a large skillet over medium heat. Add the onions and garlic and sauté until the onions are translucent, about 2 minutes. Add the ground chicken and cook, breaking up the meat into small pieces with a spatula, until no pink remains, about 2 minutes.

3. Add the egg white mixture and cook until the mixture thickens and small curds form, scraping the bottom of the pan and whisking to keep large curds from forming, about 7 minutes. Transfer to a serving platter.

4. Garnish with the red pepper flakes and/or green onions, if desired, and serve warm.

P/E ratio **2.2** • calories **341** • fat **17g** • protein **42g** • carbs **2g** • fiber **0.2g**

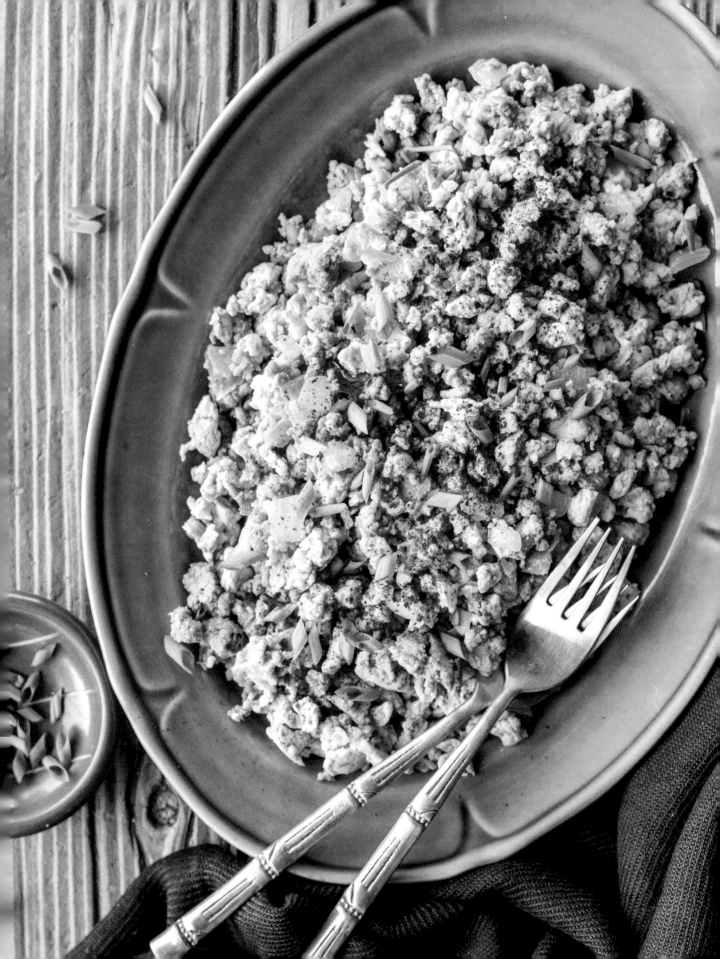

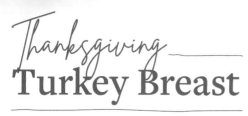

Thanksgiving
Turkey Breast

   yield: 4 servings • prep time: 7 minutes, plus 10 minutes to rest • cook time: 30 minutes

Now you can have the delicious taste of Thanksgiving at any time of the year, and the turkey doesn't take all day to cook!

3 tablespoons Dijon mustard

1 (2-pound) boneless, skinless turkey breast

1½ teaspoons fine sea salt

1 teaspoon freshly ground black pepper

1 teaspoon chopped fresh rosemary leaves

1 teaspoon chopped fresh sage

1 teaspoon chopped fresh tarragon

1 teaspoon chopped fresh thyme leaves

1. Preheat the oven to 375°F. Brush the mustard on all sides of the turkey breast.

2. Put the salt, pepper, and herbs in a small bowl and stir well. Rub the herb mixture on all sides of the turkey breast.

3. Place the turkey on a rimmed baking sheet or in a 9 by 13-inch baking dish and bake until the internal temperature reaches 162°F, about 30 minutes. Transfer to a cutting board and allow to rest until the internal temperature climbs to 165°F, about 10 minutes.

4. Cut into thick slices and serve.

P/E ratio **12.1** • calories **346** • fat **5g** • protein **69g** • carbs **1g** • fiber **0.3g**

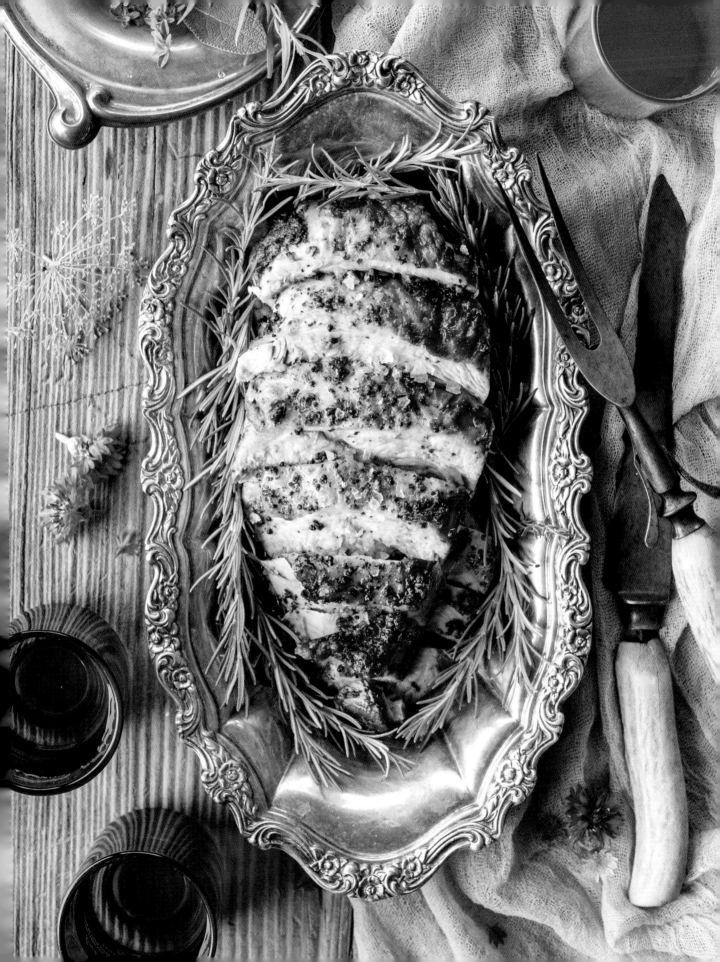

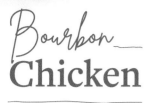

Bourbon Chicken

  yield: 4 servings • prep time: 5 minutes • cook time: 20 minutes

Although there is no bourbon in this version, this recipe makes a flavorful sticky-sweet chicken that is delicious served with Fried "Rice," or with cauliflower rice for non-PSMF days.

1 teaspoon coconut oil, lard, or tallow

2 pounds boneless, skinless chicken breasts, cut into bite-sized pieces

½ cup chicken broth

⅓ cup confectioners'-style erythritol

⅓ cup wheat-free tamari

¼ cup tomato sauce

1 tablespoon coconut vinegar or apple cider vinegar

¾ teaspoon red pepper flakes

¼ teaspoon peeled and grated fresh ginger

1 clove garlic, minced

Green onions, sliced on the diagonal, for garnish

Fried "Rice" (page 226), for serving (optional)

1. Heat the oil in a wok or large cast-iron skillet over medium-high heat. Add the chicken and stir-fry until light golden brown on all sides, about 4 minutes. Remove the chicken from the wok and set aside.

2. Add the broth, sweetener, tamari, tomato sauce, vinegar, red pepper flakes, ginger, and garlic to the wok and stir to combine. Simmer until the sauce thickens to the consistency of a loose glaze, about 10 minutes.

3. Return the chicken to the wok and simmer until the sauce forms a thick glaze coating the chicken, 5 to 10 minutes.

4. Garnish with green onions. Serve with fried "rice," if desired.

P/E ratio **5.9** • calories **316** • fat **7g** • protein **62g** • carbs **4g** • fiber **0.5g**

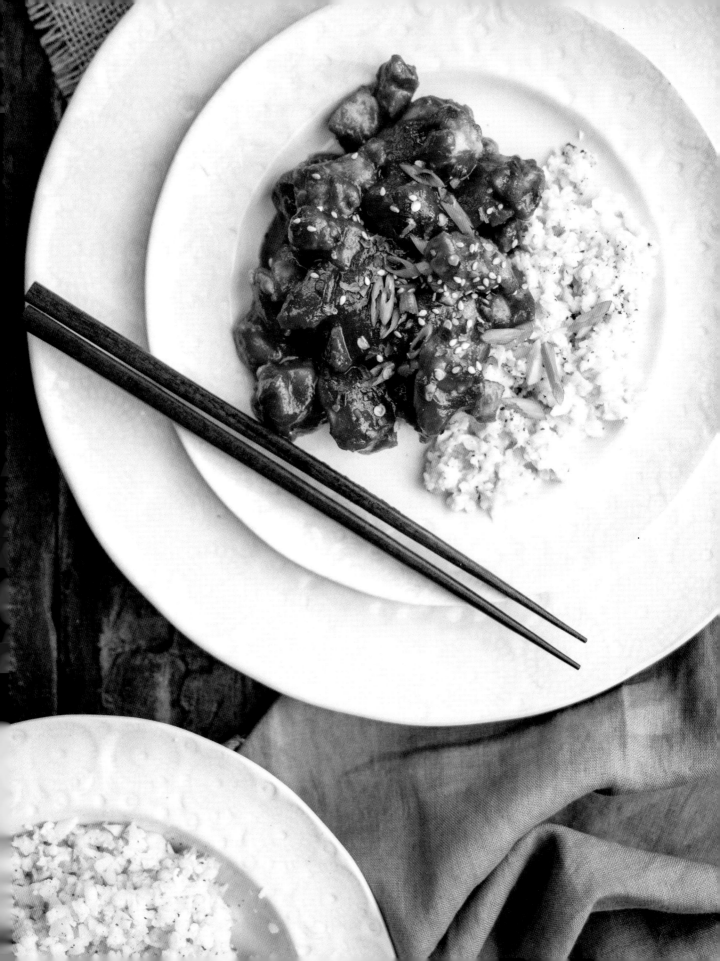

Buffalo Chicken Meatballs

  yield: 2 servings • prep time: 8 minutes • cook time: 15 minutes

My favorite hot sauce to use in this recipe is Primal Kitchen's Buffalo Sauce, but you can use any sugar-free hot sauce you like.

1 pound extra-lean ground chicken or 95% lean ground turkey

½ cup hot sauce, divided

2 large egg whites

2 tablespoons finely chopped celery

1 teaspoon fine sea salt

½ teaspoon freshly ground black pepper

Celery sticks, for serving (optional)

1. Preheat the oven to 400°F. Line a rimmed baking sheet with parchment paper.

2. In a medium-sized bowl, combine the ground chicken, ¼ cup of the hot sauce, the egg whites, celery, salt, and pepper. Form the mixture into 1¼-inch balls. (It will be easier to do this with lightly moistened hands, as the mixture is sticky.)

3. Arrange the meatballs on the prepared baking sheet and bake until golden brown, about 15 minutes. Transfer to a serving plate.

4. Pour the remaining ¼ cup of hot sauce over the meatballs and stir gently to coat. Serve warm with celery sticks, if desired.

P/E ratio **20.0** • calories **243** • fat **2g** • protein **54g** • carbs **1g** • fiber **0.3g**

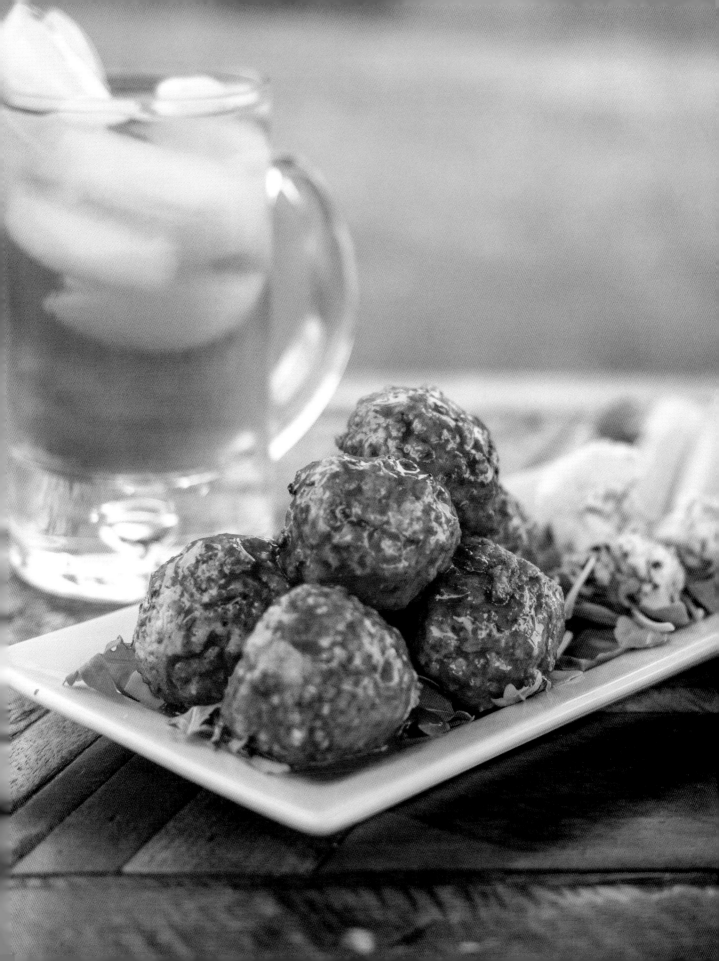

Baked Chicken Breasts with Ginger Sauce

   yield: 4 servings • prep time: 5 minutes • cook time: 22 minutes

4 (6-ounce) boneless, skinless chicken breasts

1 teaspoon fine sea salt

½ teaspoon freshly ground black pepper

Ginger Sauce:

½ cup beef or chicken broth

¼ cup peeled and grated fresh ginger

¼ cup diced yellow onions

2 cloves garlic, minced

2 tablespoons lime juice

1 teaspoon fish sauce

⅛ teaspoon liquid stevia, or more to taste

1 teaspoon fine sea salt

1. Preheat the oven to 400°F. Line a rimmed baking sheet with parchment paper.

2. Pat the chicken breasts dry with paper towels and season on both sides with the salt and pepper. Place on the prepared baking sheet and bake until the internal temperature reaches 162°F, about 22 minutes.

3. Meanwhile, make the sauce: Heat the broth in a small saucepan over medium-high heat. Add the ginger, onions, garlic, lime juice, fish sauce, stevia, and salt. Simmer until thickened slightly, about 20 minutes. Blend with an immersion blender until smooth. Taste and add more stevia, if desired. Remove from the heat and keep warm.

4. Remove the chicken from the oven and let it rest until the internal temperature reaches 165°F, 5 to 10 minutes.

5. Cut the chicken into thick slices and place in a bowl. Spoon the sauce over the chicken and serve.

P/E ratio **5.1** • calories **370** • fat **8g** • protein **72g** • carbs **7g** • fiber **1g**

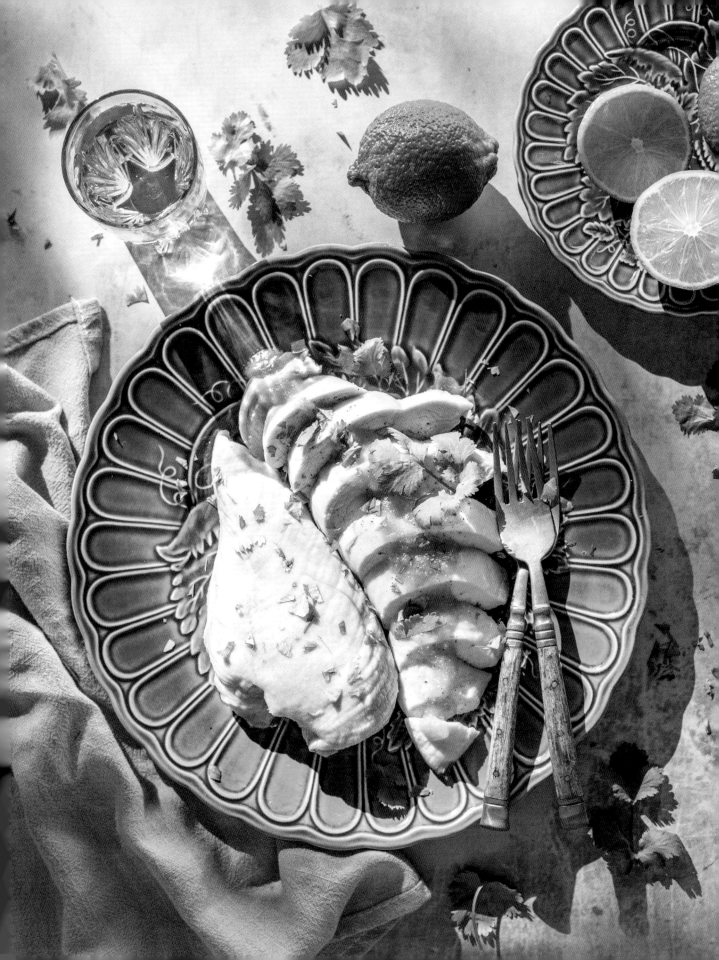

Turkey Meatloaf
with Dijon Sauce

  yield: 8 servings • prep time: 15 minutes, plus 15 minutes to rest • cook time: 45 minutes

2 pounds 95% lean ground turkey

1 cup diced button mushrooms

¼ cup diced yellow onions

2 tablespoons Dijon mustard

1 large egg white

3 teaspoons fine sea salt

½ teaspoon freshly ground black pepper

Dijon Sauce:

½ cup chicken or beef broth

¼ cup Dijon mustard

3 tablespoons lemon juice

2 cloves garlic, minced

1 teaspoon dried oregano leaves

1 teaspoon dried thyme leaves

1. Preheat the oven to 350°F. Line a 9 by 5-inch loaf pan with parchment paper.

2. Put the ground turkey, mushrooms, onions, mustard, egg white, salt, and pepper in a large bowl. Use your hands to combine the ingredients well. Press the mixture into the prepared pan. Bake until the internal temperature of the meatloaf reaches 165°F, 45 to 55 minutes.

3. Meanwhile, make the sauce: Put all of the sauce ingredients in a small saucepan. Bring to a simmer over medium-high heat and continue simmering until the sauce has reduced and thickened, about 10 minutes.

4. Remove the meatloaf from the oven and allow to rest for 15 minutes.

5. Cut the meatloaf into slices and serve with the sauce.

P/E ratio **7.0** • calories **330** • fat **6g** • protein **56g** • carbs **3g** • fiber **1g**

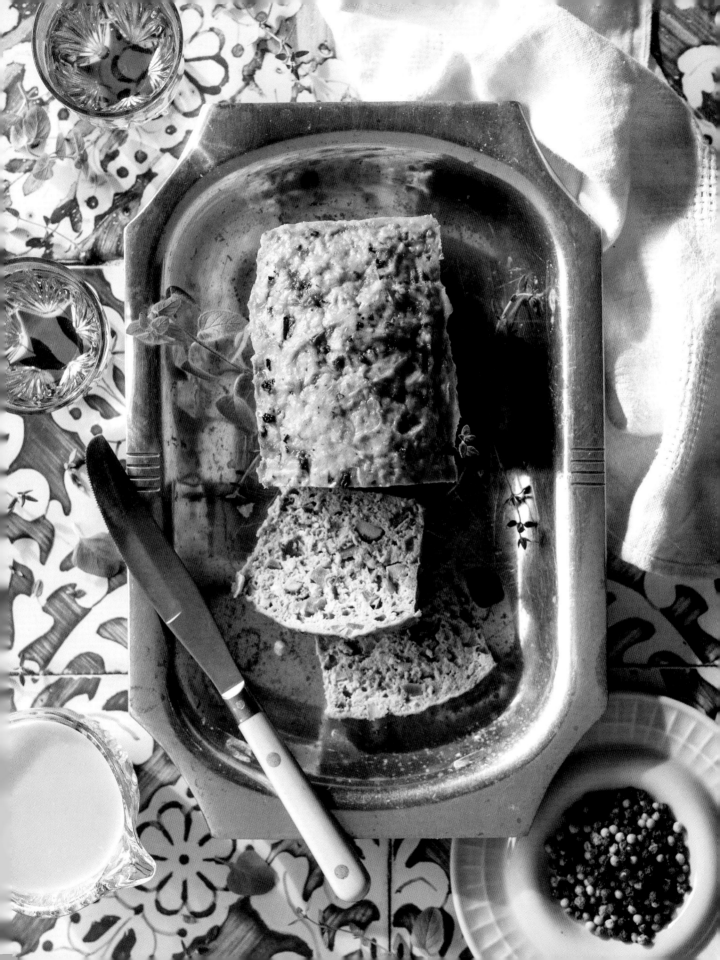

Slow Cooker
Doro Wat

  yield: 8 servings • prep time: 8 minutes • cook time: 8 to 14 hours

When we were in Ethiopia, one of the foods we ate all the time was doro wat. It is a traditional dish made with chicken, hard-boiled eggs, and lots of onions. The trick is the spice blend used, called berbere, which you can find in most health-food stores or online. I just ordered another canister because my boys love this dish. This is a very special dish to my family!

Traditional Ethiopian doro wat is very spicy. If you like spice and want a traditional doro wat, use 3 tablespoons of berbere. However, if you are like me and prefer it milder, use just 1 tablespoon.

1 large yellow onion, finely chopped

2 cloves garlic, minced

¼ cup chicken broth

2 tablespoons coconut oil, lard, or tallow

1 to 3 tablespoons berbere

1 teaspoon fine sea salt

8 (6-ounce) boneless, skinless chicken breasts

8 large hard-boiled eggs, halved

Fresh cilantro leaves, for garnish (optional)

Protein-Sparing Bread (page 270), for serving (optional)

1. Put the onion, garlic, broth, oil, berbere, and salt in a 6-quart slow cooker. Cover and cook on low until the onions are caramelized, 4 to 8 hours.

2. Add the chicken to the slow cooker and continue to cook until the meat is very tender, another 4 to 6 hours.

3. Place a chicken breast in each of eight serving bowls. Ladle the sauce in the slow cooker over the chicken. Halve the eggs and place them to one side. Garnish with cilantro, if using, and serve with Protein-Sparing Bread, if desired.

note: To make this recipe in an Instant Pot, put the onion, garlic, broth, oil, berbere, and salt in a 6-quart Instant Pot. Seal and press Manual to cook for 10 minutes. After 10 minutes, press Natural Release. Stir well. Add the chicken breasts. Seal and press Manual to cook for another 15 minutes. Press Natural Release. Stir in the hard-boiled eggs and serve as described in step 3 above.

P/E ratio **2.5** • calories **430** • fat **21g** • protein **57g** • carbs **2g** • fiber **0.3g**

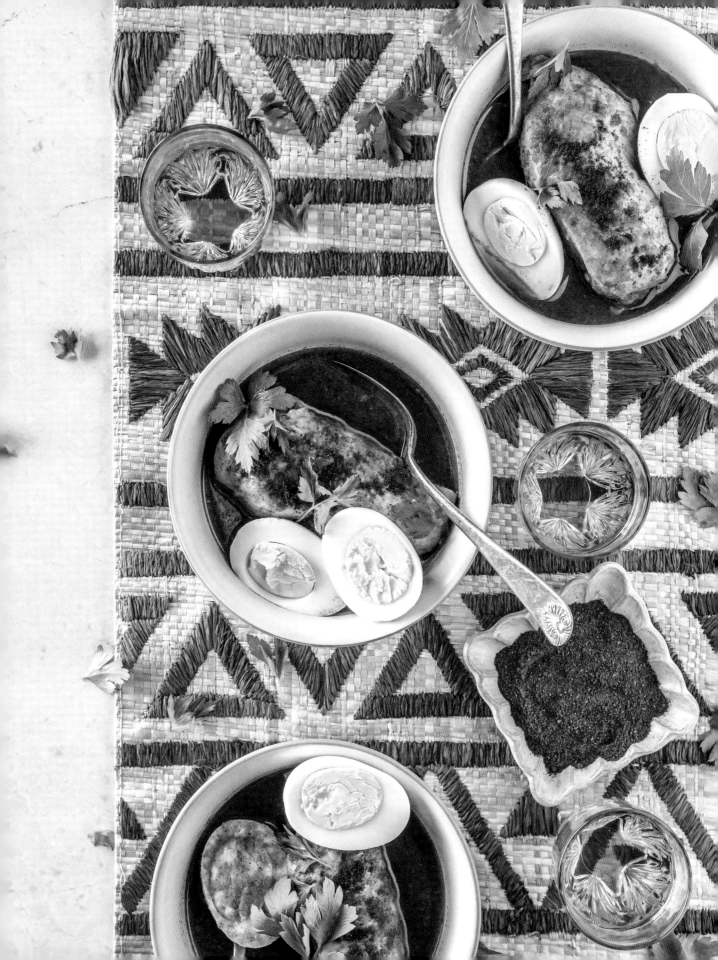

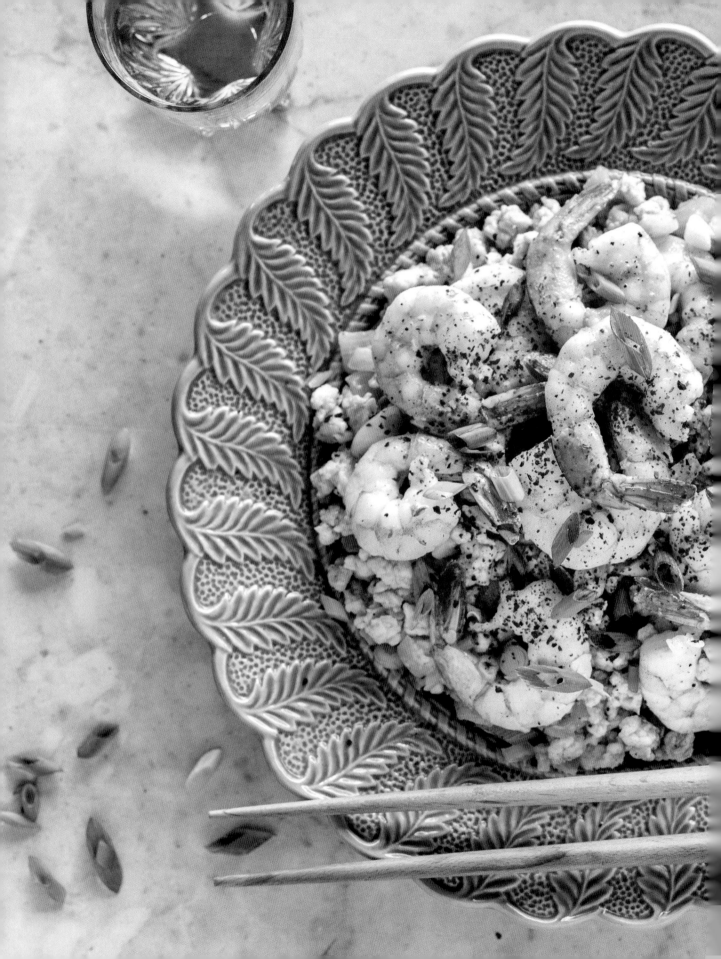

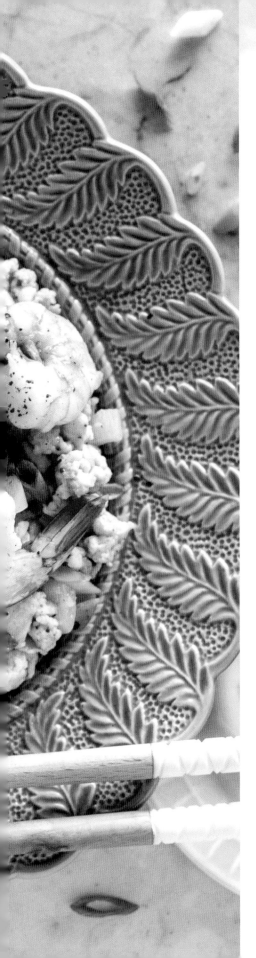

Main Dishes
Seafood

Shrimp and Grits / 160

Popovers with Tuna Salad / 162

Broiled Cod with Tartar Sauce / 164

Boiled Crab Legs with Spicy Mustard Sauce / 166

Shrimp Curry / 168

Tuna Salad with Dijon Mustard / 170

Grilled Crab Legs / 171

Surf and Turf with Carolina BBQ Sauce / 172

Broiled Shrimp with Cilantro Lime Sauce / 174

Fried Soft-Shell Crabs / 176

Poached Lobster Tails / 177

Adobo-Style Shrimp / 178

Shrimp Fried "Rice" / 180

Salt-Crusted Fish / 182

Mexican-Inspired Shrimp Kabobs / 184

Tuna Salad Dutch Baby / 186

Salmon Ceviche / 188

Basil Shrimp Ceviche / 190

Sorrento Fish / 192

Peel-and-Eat Ginger-Lime Shrimp / 194

Halibut with Ginger Sauce / 196

Baked Garlic and Herb Lobster Tails / 198

Broiled Scallops / 200

Mediterranean-Style Grilled Swordfish / 202

Shrimp Scampi / 204

Salmon in Ramen Broth / 206

Shrimp and Grits

  yield: 2 servings • prep time: 2 minutes • cook time: 10 minutes

8 large egg whites

1 cup unsweetened almond milk or cashew milk

1½ teaspoons fine sea salt, divided

2 teaspoons coconut oil (preferably butter-flavored), divided

12 precooked frozen large shrimp, thawed

Chopped fresh herbs, such as parsley or cilantro, for garnish (optional)

1. Make the grits: In a medium-sized bowl, whisk together the egg whites, milk, and 1 teaspoon of the salt. Melt 1 teaspoon of the oil in a large saucepan over medium heat. Add the egg white mixture and cook, whisking, until the mixture thickens and small curds form, about 8 minutes. Remove from the heat and keep warm.

2. Heat the remaining 1 teaspoon of oil in a large skillet over high heat. When the oil is hot, season the shrimp with the remaining ½ teaspoon of salt and sear on both sides until lightly browned and heated through, about 20 seconds per side.

3. Divide the grits between two serving bowls and top with the seared shrimp. Garnish with herbs, if desired, and serve immediately.

P/E ratio **4.8** • calories **191** • fat **6g** • protein **32g** • carbs **1g** • fiber **0.3g**

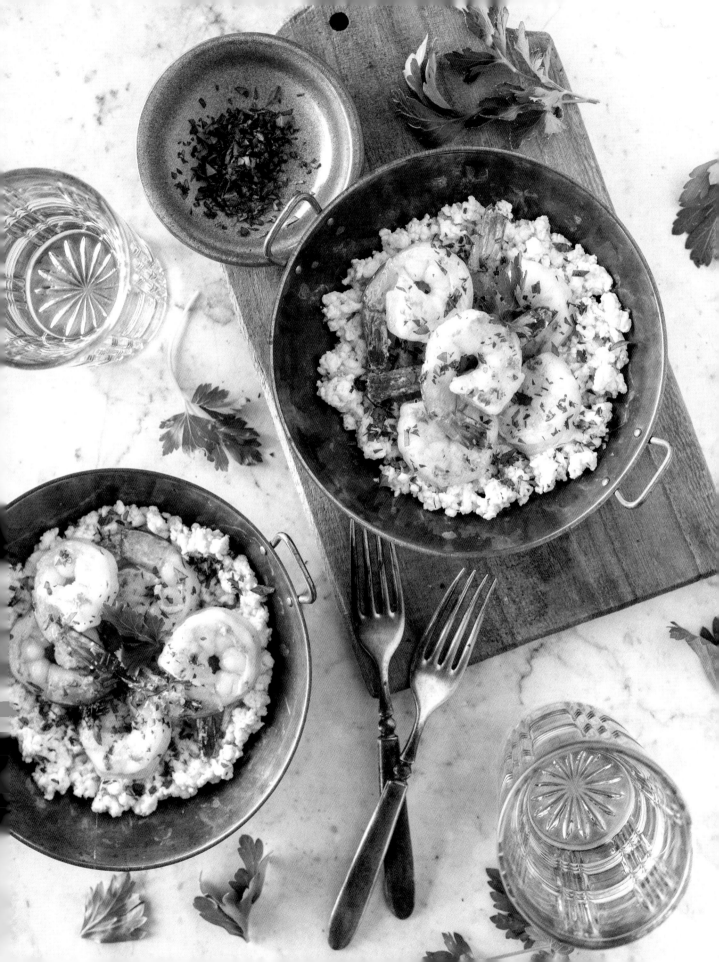

Popovers
with Tuna Salad

 yield: 4 servings • prep time: 7 minutes (not including time to make mayo) • cook time: 25 minutes

It's important that you use egg white protein powder in this recipe. Other kinds of protein powder, like whey, will not work.

Popovers:

½ cup unflavored egg white protein powder

¼ cup coconut oil, melted, plus 8 teaspoons for greasing the tins

2 cups unsweetened almond milk or cashew milk

4 large eggs

1 teaspoon baking powder

½ teaspoon fine sea salt

Tuna Salad:

2 (5-ounce) cans solid white tuna in water, drained and flaked

3 tablespoons prepared yellow mustard or Dijon mustard

2 tablespoons Mayo (page 269)

¼ teaspoon celery salt or fine sea salt

½ teaspoon freshly ground black pepper

Special Equipment:

Popover tin with at least 8 wells

1. Preheat the oven to 425°F. Put a popover tin in the hot oven for about 8 minutes.

2. Meanwhile, whisk together the protein powder, oil, milk, eggs, baking powder, and salt in a medium-sized bowl (or blend in a blender) until frothy.

3. Carefully remove the hot tin from the oven. Place 1 teaspoon of oil in each of 8 wells and divide the batter evenly among the wells, filling them about two-thirds full. Bake for 20 minutes.

4. Poke a hole in each popover with a toothpick to release moisture so they don't deflate. Reduce the oven temperature to 325°F and bake until the popovers are golden and puffed, 5 to 7 minutes more.

5. Meanwhile, make the tuna salad: Put the tuna, mustard, mayo, celery salt, and pepper in a medium-sized bowl and stir to combine well.

6. Remove the popovers from the oven and allow to cool a bit. Serve with the tuna salad on the side. You can also slice the popovers in half and fill them with the tuna salad.

P/E ratio **1.3** • calories **378** • fat **26g** • protein **34g** • carbs **1g** • fiber **0.3g**

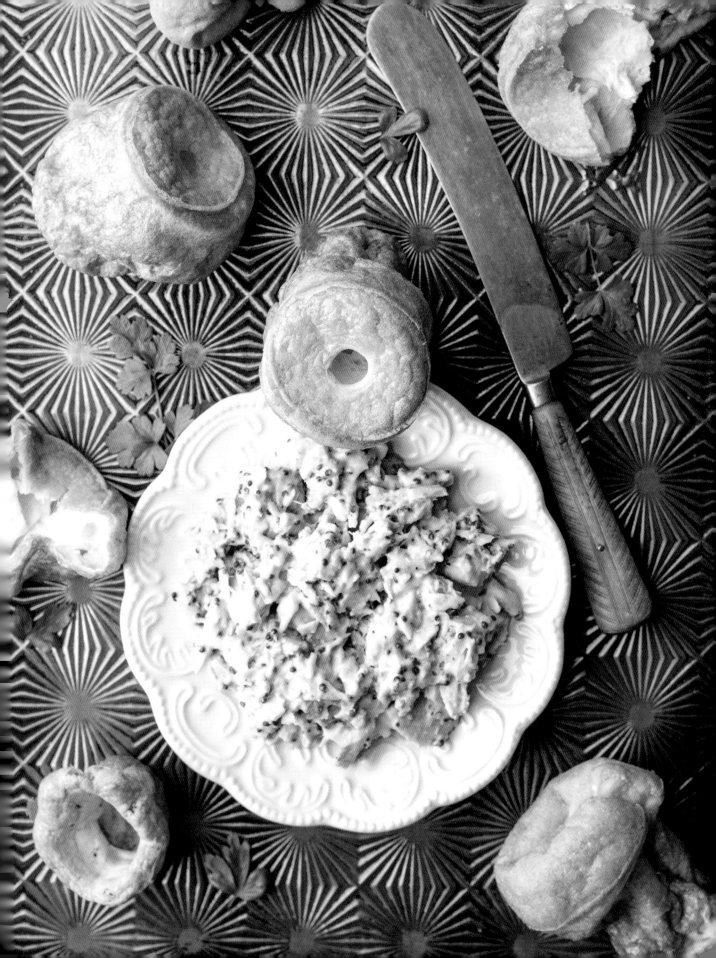

Broiled Cod
with Tartar Sauce

  yield: 1 serving • prep time: 10 minutes (not including time to make mayo) • cook time: 10 minutes

2 (6-ounce) cod fillets or other white fish fillets

½ teaspoon garlic powder

½ teaspoon smoked paprika

½ teaspoon fine sea salt

½ teaspoon freshly ground black pepper

Tartar Sauce (*makes ¾ cup*):

½ cup Mayo (page 269)

2 tablespoons dill pickle juice

2 tablespoons finely chopped dill pickles

Fresh parsley leaves, for garnish (optional)

Lemon wedges, for serving (optional)

1. Place an oven rack 6 inches below the heating element (usually this means the second rack from the top of the oven) and turn the broiler to high (500°F). Line a rimmed baking sheet with parchment paper.

2. Place the cod fillets on the prepared baking sheet and season with the garlic powder, paprika, salt, and pepper. Broil until the fish flakes easily with a fork, about 10 minutes.

3. While the fish is baking, make the tartar sauce: Put all of the ingredients in a bowl and stir well to combine.

4. Plate the fish. Top with 1½ tablespoons of the tartar sauce and garnish with parsley, if desired. Serve with lemon wedges to squeeze over the fish, if using. Store the leftover tartar sauce in an airtight container in the refrigerator for up to 6 days.

P/E ratio **5.6** • calories **457** • fat **13g** • protein **78g** • carbs **2g** • fiber **1g**

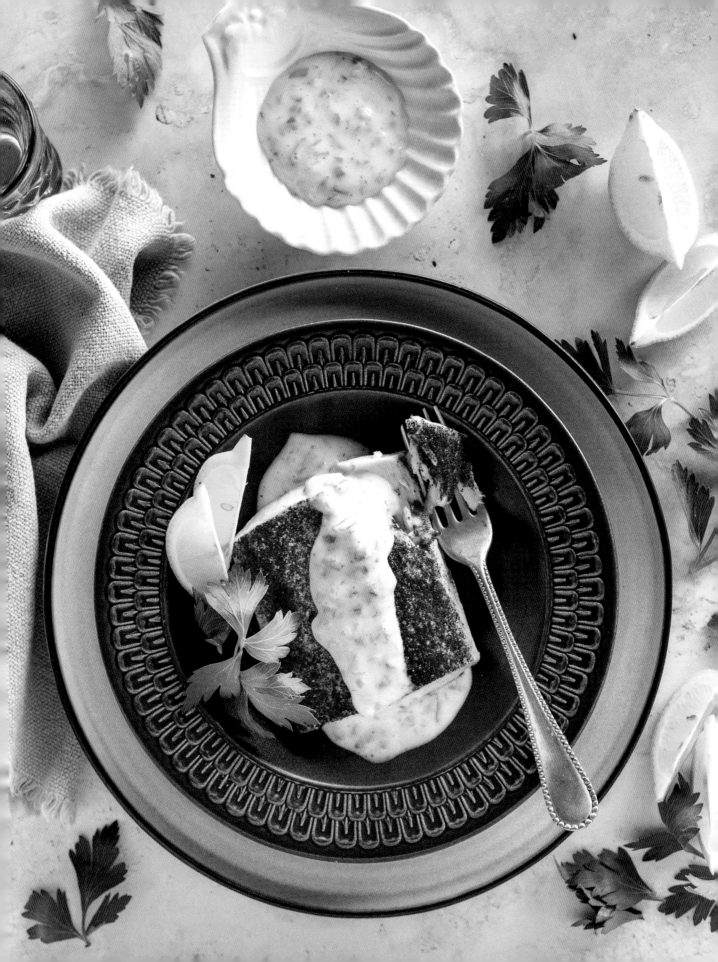

Boiled Crab Legs
with Spicy Mustard Sauce

  yield: 4 servings • prep time: 5 minutes (not including time to make mayo) • cook time: 3 minutes

I love this recipe because it's so quick and easy. Crab legs are sold already cooked, so all you have to do to pull this dish together is make the tasty sauce while warming up the crab legs.

2 tablespoons fine sea salt

12 frozen Alaskan king crab legs, thawed

Sauce:

½ cup Dijon mustard

2 tablespoons Mayo (page 269)

1 tablespoon prepared horseradish

2 teaspoons lime or lemon juice

2 or 3 drops hot sauce

⅛ teaspoon fine sea salt

For Garnish (optional):

Lime wedges

Chopped fresh parsley leaves

1. Prepare the crab legs: Fill a stockpot about two-thirds full with water and bring to a boil over high heat. Stir in the salt, add the crab legs, and boil until warmed through, about 3 minutes. Drain well.

2. Make the sauce: Put the mustard, mayo, horseradish, lime juice, hot sauce, and salt in a small mixing bowl. Stir well to combine, then transfer to a small serving bowl.

3. Place the crab legs on a platter with the bowl of mustard sauce on the side. Garnish with lime wedges and/or parsley, if desired. Serve warm, or chill and serve cold.

P/E ratio **8.1** • calories **374** • fat **8g** • protein **71g** • carbs **1g** • fiber **0.2g**

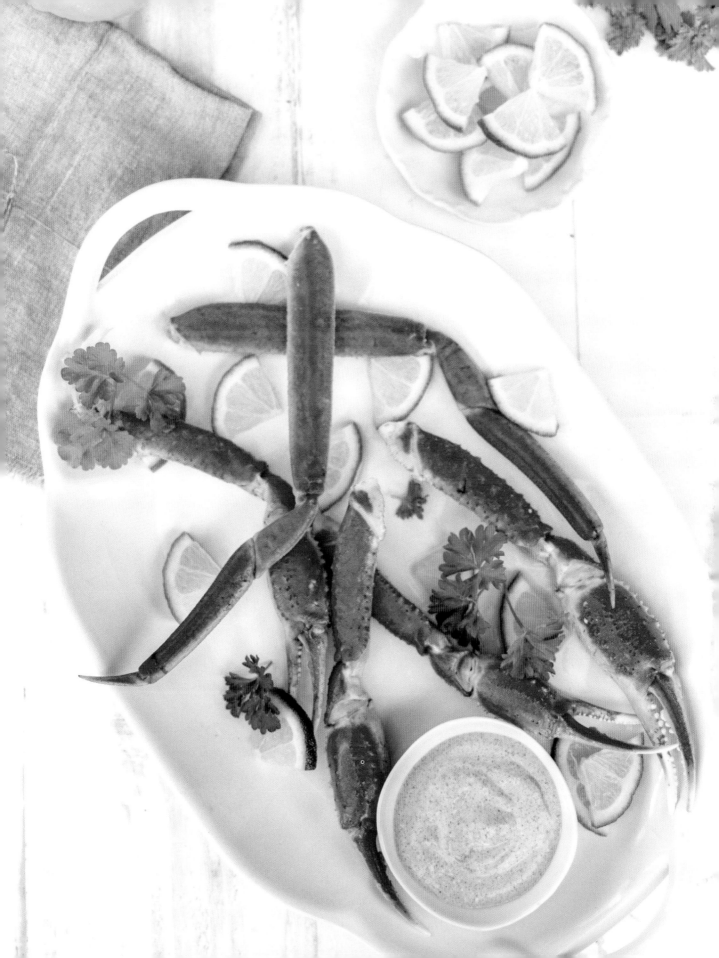

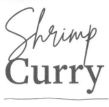

Shrimp Curry

    yield: 8 servings • prep time: 8 minutes • cook time: 10 minutes

This dish features two main seasoning ingredients: garam masala, which is a wonderful blend of spices common in Indian curries, and Thai yellow curry paste, which is packed with fresh aromatics and dried spices. Both can be found in many grocery stores or online.

¼ cup coconut oil

½ cup diced yellow onions

6 cloves garlic, minced

2 tablespoons peeled and grated fresh ginger

2 pounds medium-sized shrimp, peeled and deveined

2 teaspoons fine sea salt

¼ cup chicken broth

3 tablespoons garam masala

2 tablespoons Thai yellow curry paste

1 tablespoon turmeric powder

1 tablespoon lime juice

Fried "Rice" (page 226), for serving (optional)

For Garnish:

Lime slices

Fresh cilantro leaves

Green onions, sliced on the diagonal

1. Heat the oil in a large cast-iron skillet over medium-high heat. Add the onions and sauté until soft, about 3 minutes. Add the garlic and ginger and sauté for another 2 minutes.

2. Add the shrimp and salt to the skillet and cook until firm and opaque, about 2 minutes.

3. Add the broth, garam masala, curry paste, and turmeric powder to the pan. Stir to combine; simmer for 2 minutes. Stir in the lime juice and remove the pan from the heat.

4. Serve over fried "rice," if desired, and garnish with lime slices, cilantro leaves, and green onions.

P/E ratio **1.2** • calories **252** • fat **15g** • protein **24g** • carbs **6g** • fiber **1g**

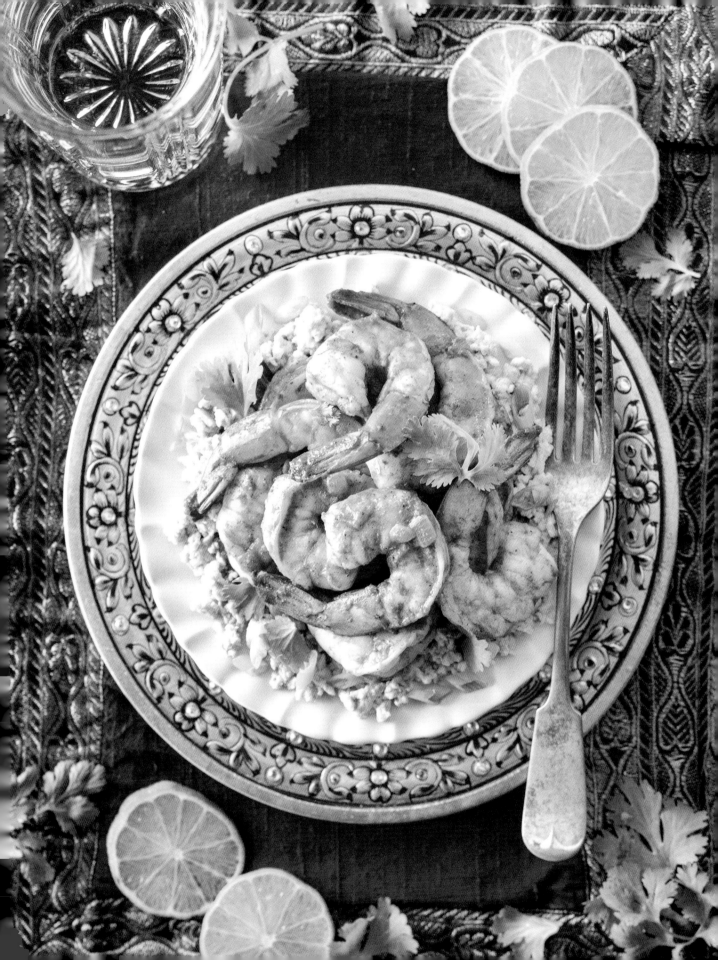

Tuna Salad
with Dijon Mustard

  yield: 2 servings • prep time: 5 minutes (not including time to make mayo)

This tuna salad is great on its own or as a sandwich filling, using Protein-Sparing Bread (page 270).

2 (5-ounce) cans solid white tuna in water, drained and flaked

¼ cup Dijon mustard

2 tablespoons Mayo (page 269)

¼ teaspoon celery salt or fine sea salt

⅛ teaspoon freshly ground black pepper

1. Put the tuna, mustard, mayo, celery salt, and pepper in a medium-sized bowl and stir to combine well. Taste and adjust the seasoning to your liking.

2. Store in an airtight container in the refrigerator for up to 4 days.

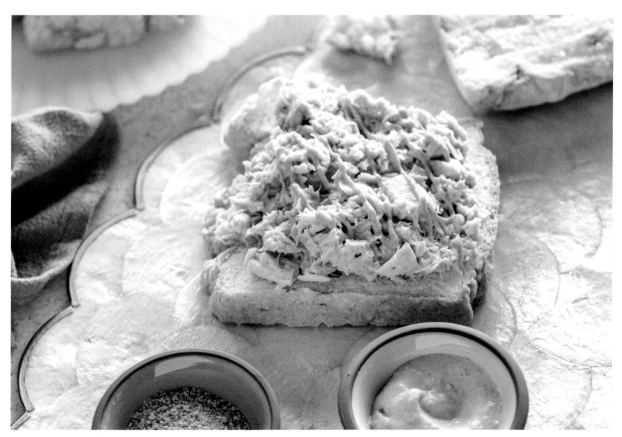

P/E ratio **2.2** • calories **295** • fat **15g** • protein **37g** • carbs **2g** • fiber **0g**

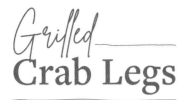
Grilled Crab Legs

    yield: 4 servings • prep time: 5 minutes • cook time: 10 minutes

4 pounds frozen king crab legs, thawed and rinsed

1. Heat the grill to medium-high heat.

2. Arrange the crab legs on the grill grates. Cover and cook for 5 minutes; flip and cook until heated through, about 5 minutes longer.

3. To deshell the crab legs, hold one with a mitted or gloved hand and, with a sharp paring knife in the other hand, cut a slit along the length of the leg and pull the meat out. Repeat with the remaining crab legs. Arrange the crabmeat on a serving platter and enjoy.

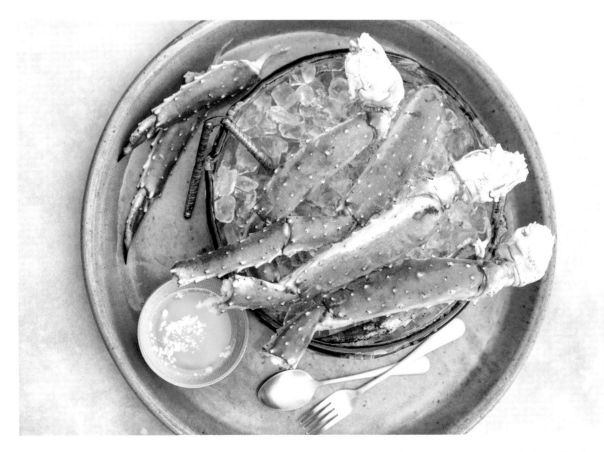

P/E ratio 12.6 • calories 440 • fat 7g • protein 88g • carbs 0g • fiber 0g   The Protein-Sparing Modified Fast Method

Surf and Turf
with Carolina BBQ Sauce

   yield: 2 servings • prep time: 5 minutes, plus 15 minutes to marinate and 10 minutes to rest (not including time to make BBQ sauce) • cook time: 15 minutes

2 (3-ounce) filet mignons

1½ teaspoons fine sea salt

¾ teaspoon freshly ground black pepper

2 tablespoons coconut oil, lard, tallow, or bacon fat, for frying

4 jumbo prawns or jumbo shrimp, shell-on, butterflied, and deveined

¼ cup Carolina BBQ Sauce (page 267), for serving

1. Season the steaks on all sides with the salt and pepper. Let them sit at room temperature for 15 minutes.

2. Heat a medium-sized cast-iron skillet over medium-high heat. Melt the oil in the pan, then add the steaks. Cook for 4 minutes per side for medium-rare. Remove the filets from the skillet and allow to rest for 10 minutes. Keep the skillet on the burner.

3. While the filets are resting, add the prawns to the skillet and cook until the shells have turned pink and the meat is firm and opaque, about 3 minutes per side.

4. Plate the steaks. Top each with 2 prawns and serve with the BBQ sauce.

P/E ratio **1.3** • calories **316** • fat **22g** • protein **29g** • carbs **2g** • fiber **1g**

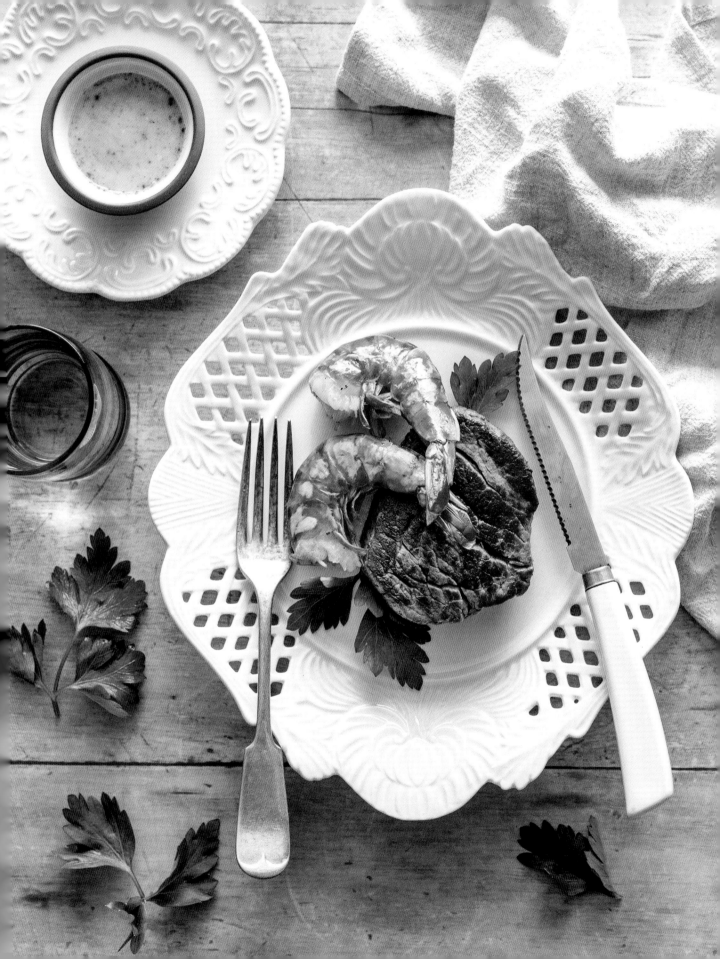

Broiled Shrimp
with Cilantro Lime Sauce

   yield: 4 servings • prep time: 5 minutes (not including time to make sauce) • cook time: 15 minutes

2 tablespoons melted coconut oil, lard, or tallow

1 tablespoon lime or lemon juice

1 teaspoon fine sea salt

1 teaspoon smoked paprika

1 clove garlic, minced

8 ounces medium-sized shrimp, peeled and deveined

Fresh cilantro leaves, for garnish (optional)

¼ cup Cilantro Lime Sauce (page 268), for serving

1. Place an oven rack 6 inches below the heating element (usually this means the second rack from the top of the oven). Turn the broiler to high (500°F). Line a rimmed baking sheet with parchment paper.

2. Put the oil, lime juice, salt, paprika, and garlic in a large bowl. Stir well to combine. Add the shrimp and stir well to coat.

3. Arrange the shrimp on the prepared baking sheet and broil until opaque and slightly charred, about 5 minutes.

4. Garnish the shrimp with cilantro leaves, if using, and serve with the cilantro lime sauce.

P/E ratio **2.0** • calories **274** • fat **14g** • protein **35g** • carbs **4g** • fiber **0.4g**

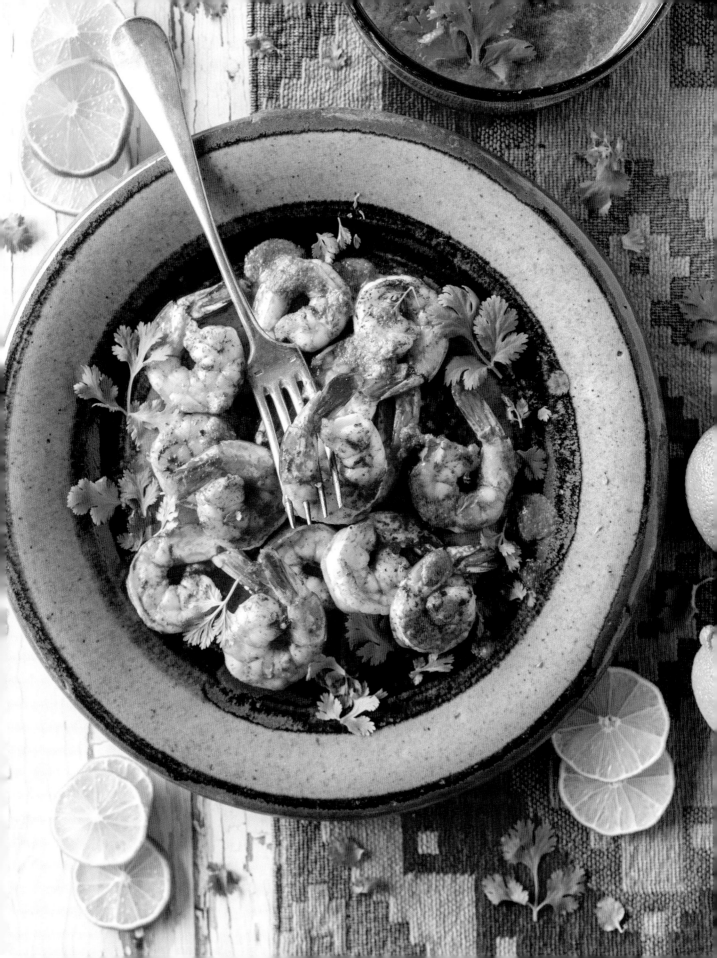

Fried
Soft-Shell Crabs

  yield: 2 servings • prep time: 8 minutes (not including time to make sauce) • cook time: 8 minutes

2 large eggs

½ cup pork rind crumbs

8 soft-shell crabs

½ cup coconut oil, lard, or tallow

¼ cup Carolina BBQ Sauce (page 267), for serving

1. Crack the eggs into a large shallow dish and beat with a fork just until combined. Put the pork rind crumbs in another large shallow dish.

2. Dip a crab in the beaten eggs and shake off the excess, then gently dredge it in the pork rind crumbs. Use your hands to pat the crumbs onto the crab, making sure it is thoroughly coated. Repeat with the remaining crabs.

3. Heat the oil in a large cast-iron skillet over medium-high heat. Line a plate with paper towels.

4. When the oil is hot, fry the crabs in batches so as not to overcrowd the pan. Cook until golden brown on both sides, about 2 minutes per side. Transfer to the paper towel–lined plate to drain.

5. Serve immediately with the BBQ sauce.

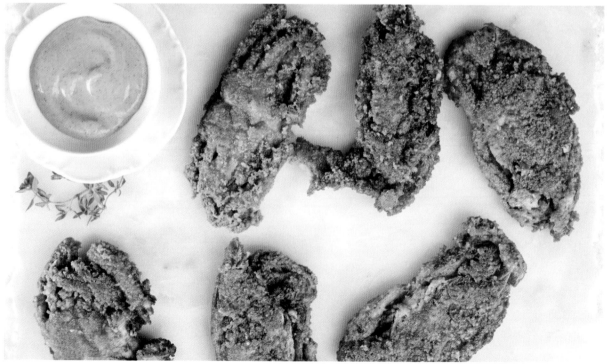

P/E ratio **4.0** • calories **388** • fat **14g** • protein **60g** • carbs **2g** • fiber **1g**

Poached
Lobster Tails

   yield: 1 serving • prep time: 5 minutes (not including time to make sauce) • cook time: 6 minutes

2 tablespoons fine sea salt

2 (4-ounce) frozen lobster tails, thawed

Carolina BBQ Sauce (page 267) or Dijon Vinaigrette (page 266), for serving (optional)

1. Fill a medium-sized saucepan halfway with water and bring to a boil over high heat.

2. Stir in the salt, then gently lower the lobster tails into the pan, adding more water to cover them, if necessary. Once the water resumes boiling, reduce the heat and simmer, uncovered, until the meat is completely opaque and the internal temperature reaches 140°F, 6 to 8 minutes. Remove the lobster tails from the saucepan and shake off excess moisture.

3. Serve immediately with BBQ sauce or vinaigrette, if desired.

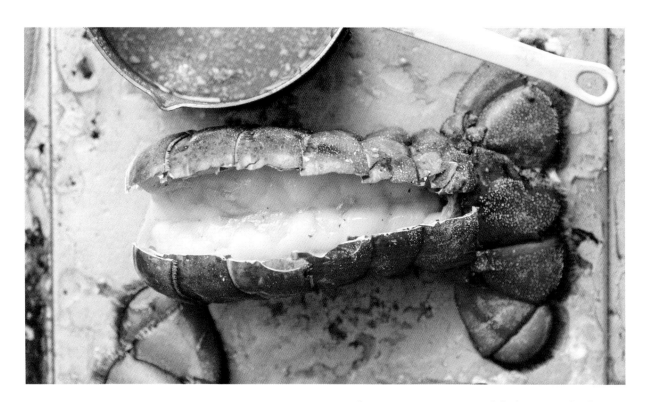

P/E ratio 16.0 • calories 225 • fat 3g • protein 48g • carbs 0g • fiber 0g   The Protein-Sparing Modified Fast Method   177

Adobo-Style Shrimp

yield: 2 servings • prep time: 4 minutes plus 2 hours for marinating • cook time: 5 minutes

Adobo is a cooking technique in the Philippines. The most traditional and widely known version features stewed meat seasoned with garlic, vinegar, soy sauce, and black pepper. I think the classic flavor of adobo goes very well with shrimp, so I have applied it to this simple shrimp stir-fry.

1 pound medium-sized shrimp, peeled and deveined

¼ cup coconut vinegar

¼ cup wheat-free tamari

2 tablespoons lime juice

1 teaspoon fish sauce

2 cloves garlic, minced

2 tablespoons freshly ground black pepper

1 teaspoon fine sea salt

2 tablespoons coconut oil, lard, or tallow

Fresh cilantro leaves, for garnish (optional)

Fried "Rice" (page 226), for serving (optional)

1. Place the shrimp in a large bowl. Add the vinegar, tamari, lime juice, fish sauce, garlic, pepper, and salt; stir to combine.

2. Heat the oil in a wok or large cast-iron skillet over medium-high heat. Once the oil is hot, add the shrimp along with the marinade. Cook, stirring often, until the shrimp are firm and opaque, about 5 minutes. Remove the pan from the heat.

3. Garnish the shrimp with cilantro, if using, and serve with fried "rice," if desired.

P/E ratio **2.2** • calories **287** • fat **14g** • protein **39g** • carbs **4g** • fiber **0.2g**

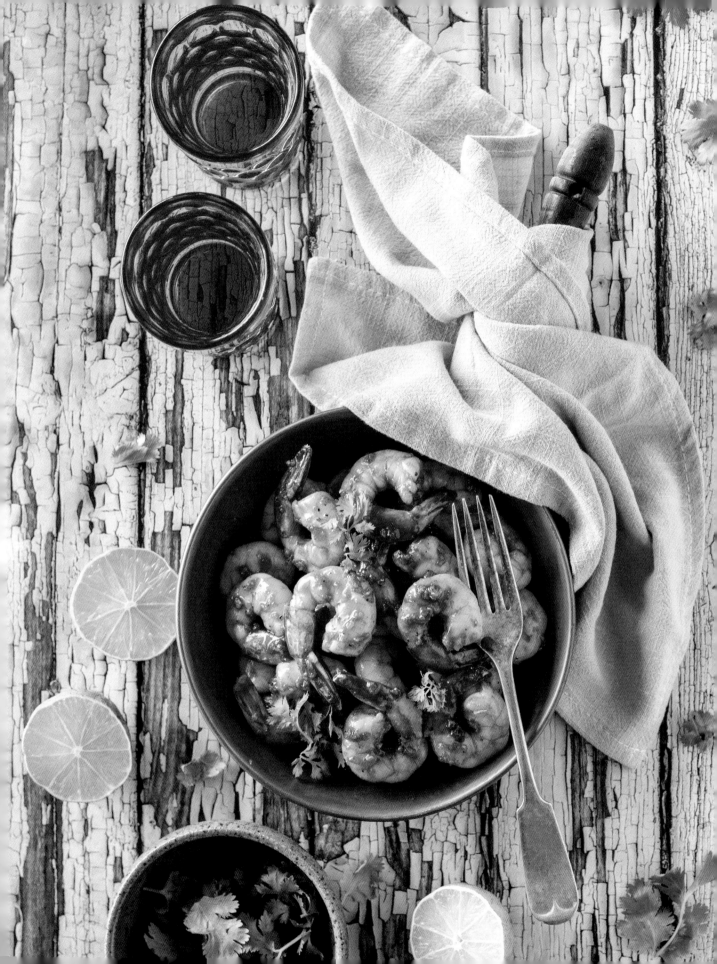

Shrimp
Fried "Rice"

  yield: 4 servings • prep time: 5 minutes • cook time: 15 minutes

12 large egg whites

2 tablespoons beef broth

1 teaspoon wheat-free tamari

1¼ teaspoons fine sea salt, divided

1 teaspoon freshly ground black pepper, divided

1 teaspoon coconut oil, lard, or tallow

¼ cup diced yellow onions

1 clove garlic, minced

1 pound large shrimp, peeled and deveined

1 teaspoon red pepper flakes

Thinly sliced green onions, for garnish (optional)

1. Put the egg whites in a large bowl. Add the broth, tamari, ½ teaspoon of the salt, and ½ teaspoon of the pepper; whisk until well combined.

2. Heat the oil in a large skillet over medium-high heat. When hot, add the onions and garlic and sauté until the onions are translucent, about 2 minutes.

3. Season the shrimp on all sides with the remaining ¾ teaspoon of salt and remaining ½ teaspoon of pepper; add to the skillet and cook for 2 minutes on each side.

4. Add the egg mixture to the pan and cook, whisking constantly, until the mixture thickens and small curds form, about 7 minutes. Remove the pan from the heat.

5. Sprinkle the red pepper flakes on top and garnish with green onions, if desired.

P/E ratio **6.8** • calories **203** • fat **3g** • protein **39g** • carbs **3g** • fiber **0.3g**

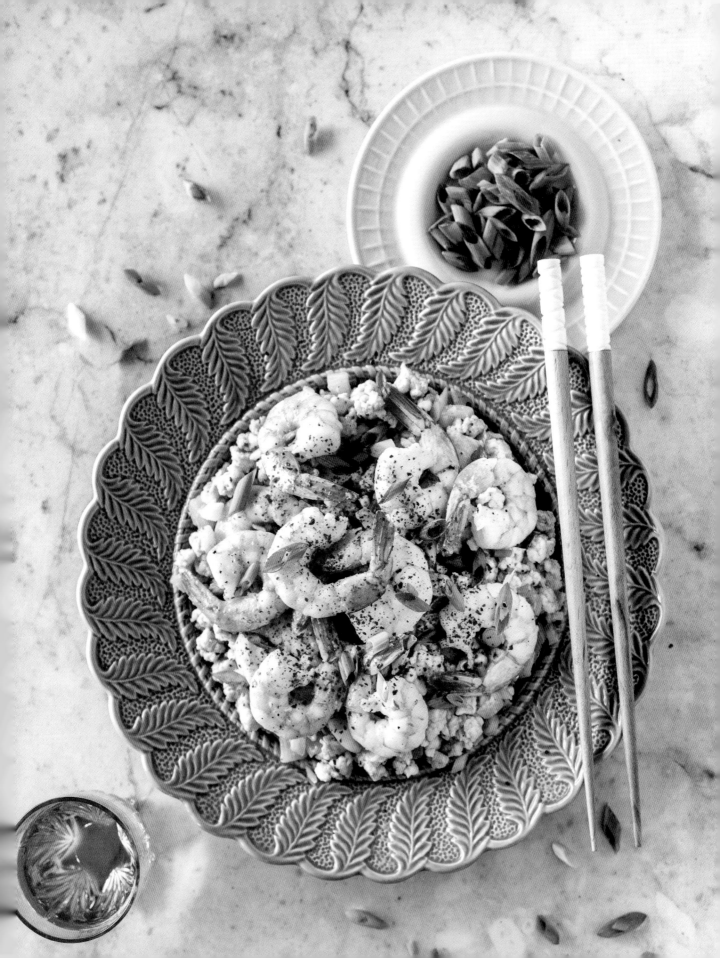

Salt-Crusted Fish

  yield: 4 servings • prep time: 10 minutes, plus 10 minutes to rest • cook time: 25 minutes

I love making this recipe for my friends and family! It is an impressive-looking dish that is very easy to make.

2 tablespoons roughly chopped fresh dill (or any leafy herb)

1 lemon, thinly sliced

1 (3-pound) whole fish, such as sea bass, red snapper, or trout, gutted, gills and fins removed

4 large egg whites

2 cups coarse sea salt

For Garnish:

2 tablespoons diced red onions

2 tablespoons capers

2 tablespoons chopped fresh dill

4 lemon slices

1. Preheat the oven to 450°F.

2. Stuff the herbs and lemon slices into the cavity of the fish. Set aside.

3. Place the egg whites in a large mixing bowl and beat with an electric hand mixer on high speed just until soft peaks form. Gently fold the salt into the whites with a rubber spatula.

4. Place a large ovenproof platter on a baking sheet. Put about ¼ cup of the egg white mixture on the platter and spread it into the size and shape of the fish. Set the fish on top and cover the fish completely with the remaining egg white mixture.

5. Bake until a meat thermometer inserted through the salt crust into the thickest part of the fish reads 125°F, about 25 minutes.

6. Let the fish rest for 10 minutes. For a dramatic presentation, place the platter on the dinner table and crack the salt crust open in front of your guests. Then fillet the fish and place on serving plates. Garnish with the onions, capers, dill, and lemon slices.

P/E ratio **2.1** • calories **390** • fat **21g** • protein **46g** • carbs **2g** • fiber **1g**

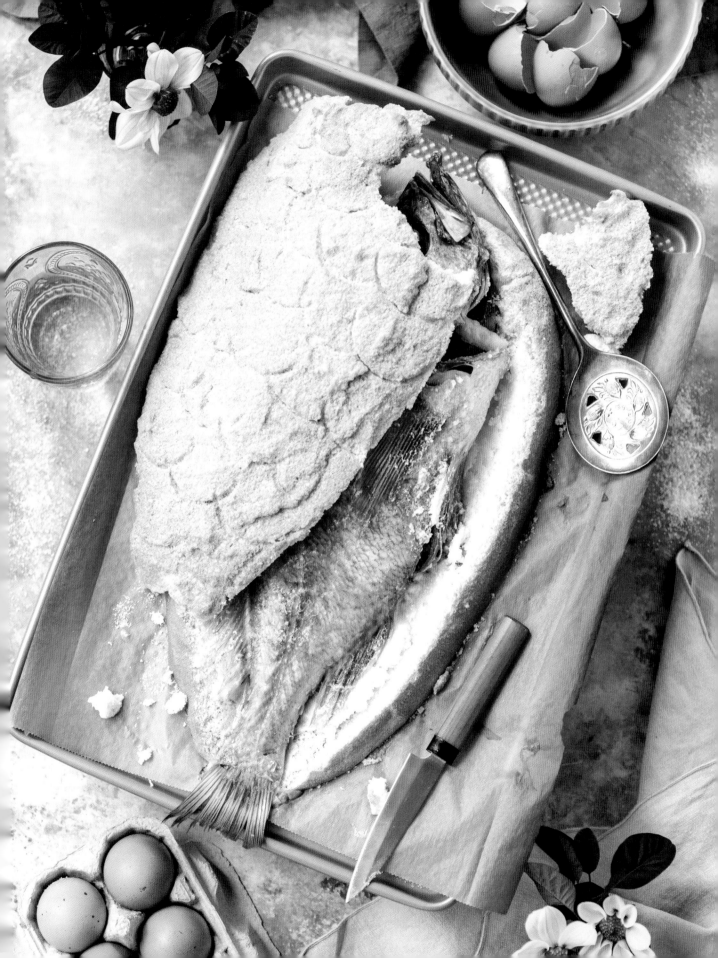

Mexican-Inspired
Shrimp Kabobs

   yield: 1 serving • prep time: 5 minutes • cook time: 6 minutes

Duck fat or coconut oil, for greasing

2 teaspoons chili powder

¼ teaspoon fine sea salt

⅛ teaspoon ground cumin

⅛ teaspoon garlic powder

⅛ teaspoon onion powder

⅛ teaspoon smoked paprika

12 medium-sized shrimp, peeled and deveined

Special Equipment:

4 skewers

1. If using wooden or bamboo skewers, soak them in water for 10 minutes.

2. Lightly grease the grates of a grill with duck fat. Heat the grill to medium-high heat.

3. In a small bowl, stir together the chili powder, salt, cumin, garlic powder, onion powder, and paprika. Put the shrimp in a medium-sized bowl and add the spice mixture to the shrimp; mix well to coat the shrimp evenly. Thread 3 shrimp onto each skewer.

4. Grill the shrimp until firm and opaque, 3 to 4 minutes per side. Remove from the grill and serve hot, or chill and serve cold.

P/E ratio **11.7** • calories **160** • fat **1g** • protein **35g** • carbs **4g** • fiber **2g**

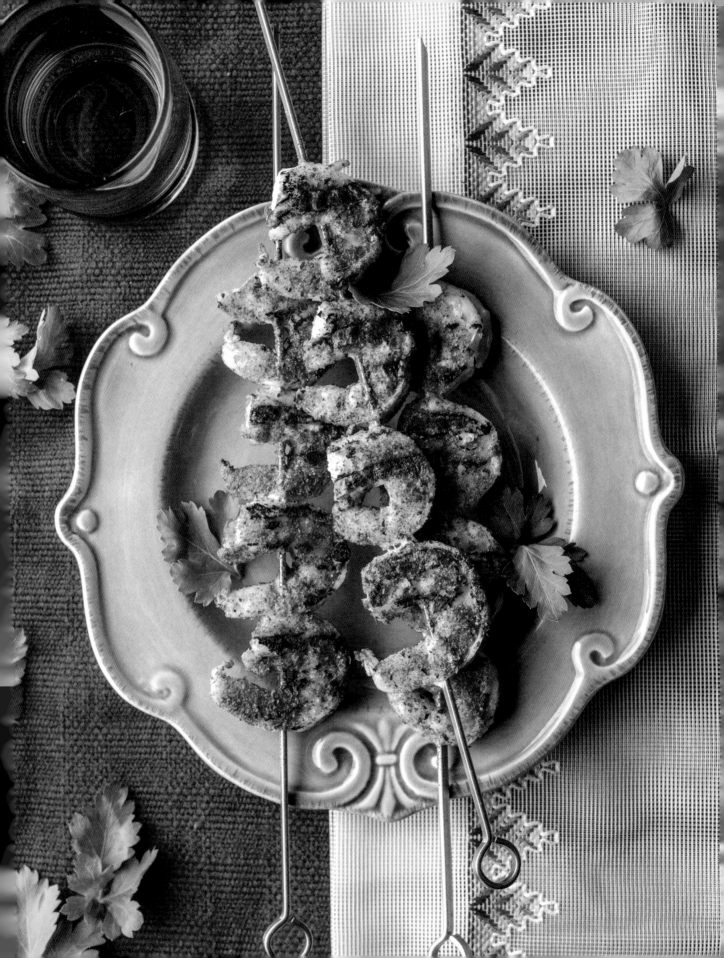

Tuna Salad
Dutch Baby

  yield: 2 servings • prep time: 5 minutes • cook time: 18 minutes

Pancake:

6 large egg whites

¾ cup beef broth

¼ cup unflavored egg white protein powder

1 teaspoon baking powder

1 teaspoon fine sea salt

Tuna Salad:

1 (5-ounce) can tuna, packed in water, drained and flaked

2 tablespoons Dijon mustard or prepared yellow mustard

Fine sea salt and freshly ground black pepper

Chopped fresh parsley leaves, for garnish (optional)

Sliced green onions, for garnish (optional)

1. Make the pancake: Place an 8-inch cast-iron skillet on a rack positioned in the middle of the oven. Set the oven to 400°F and let the skillet preheat along with the oven.

2. Put the egg whites, broth, protein powder, baking powder, and salt in a blender and blend until foamy, about 1 minute. Pour the batter into the hot skillet. Bake until the pancake is puffed and golden brown, 18 to 20 minutes.

3. Meanwhile, make the tuna salad: Put the tuna in a small bowl and flake with a fork. Stir in the mustard and season to taste with salt and pepper.

4. Remove the pancake from the oven. Spread the tuna salad on top and garnish with parsley and/or green onions, if desired. Cut into wedges and enjoy.

P/E ratio **19.5** • calories **198** • fat **1g** • protein **39g** • carbs **1g** • fiber **0g**

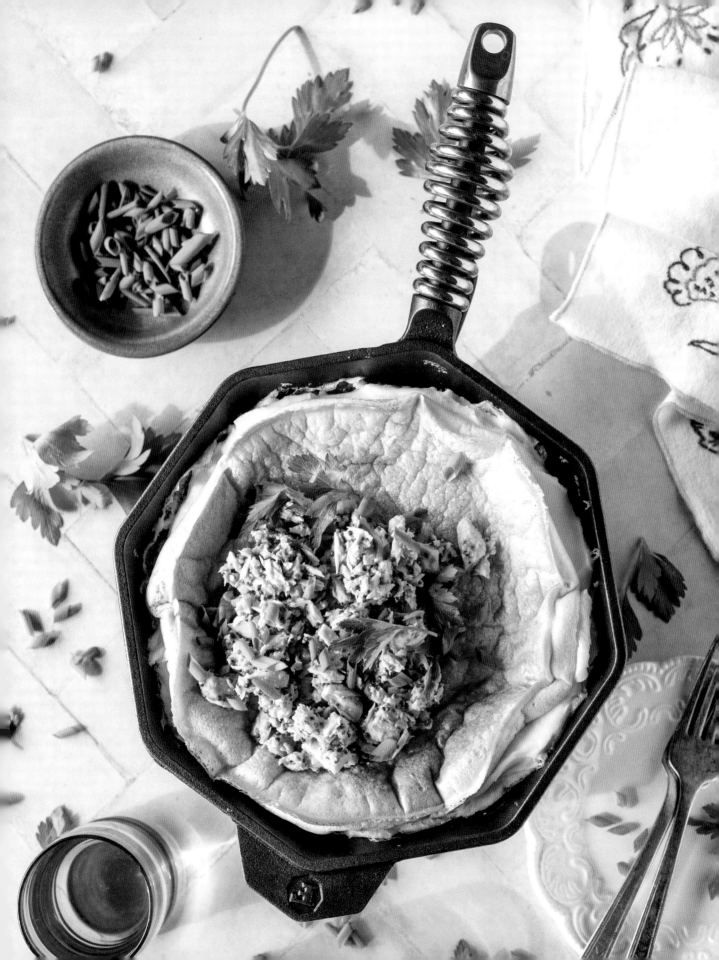

Salmon Ceviche

   yield: 2 servings • prep time: 6 minutes, plus 15 minutes to chill

Ceviche is made from fresh raw seafood cured in citrus juice. It's best, therefore, to use the freshest and highest-quality salmon you can find and to enjoy the dish immediately after it's done chilling.

5 tablespoons lime juice

1 tablespoon extra-virgin olive oil

1 clove garlic, smashed to a paste

8 ounces skinless salmon fillets, cut into ½-inch cubes

3 tablespoons diced red onions

2 tablespoons chopped fresh cilantro leaves

1 teaspoon fine sea salt

1. Combine the lime juice, oil, and garlic in a medium-sized bowl. Add the salmon, onions, cilantro, and salt. Stir well to combine.

2. Cover and refrigerate for 15 minutes before serving.

P/E ratio **3.1** • calories **156** • fat **6g** • protein **22g** • carbs **2g** • fiber **1g**

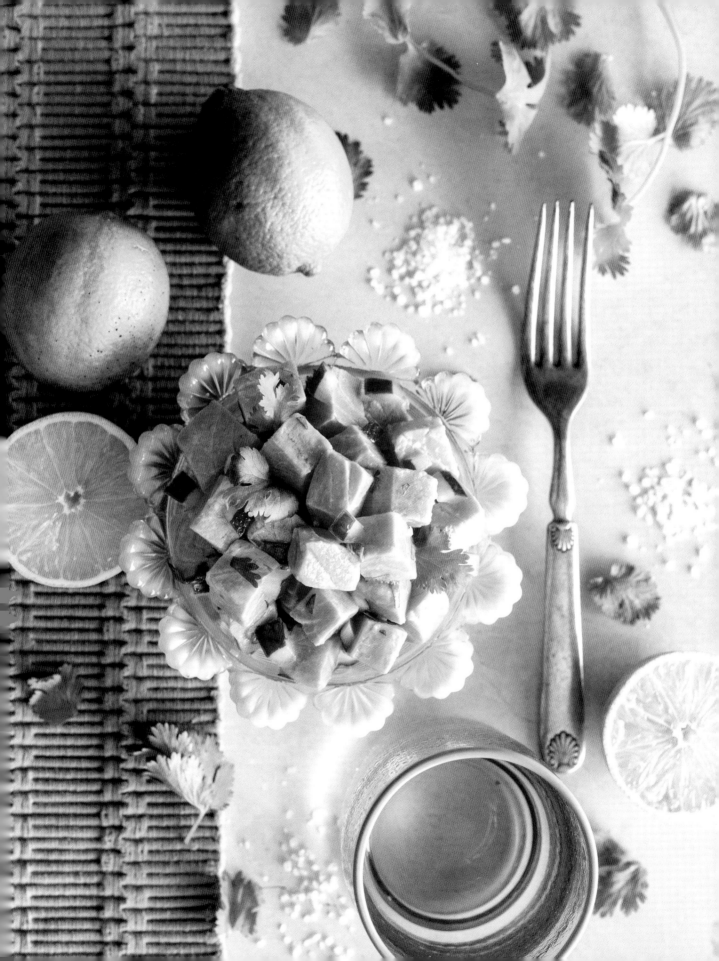

Basil
Shrimp Ceviche

   yield: 2 servings • prep time: 8 minutes, plus 15 minutes to chill

I like to use small shrimp in this recipe, but you can also use larger shrimp, deveined and cut into small pieces.

¾ cup lime juice

1 tablespoon extra-virgin olive oil

1 clove garlic, smashed into a paste

1 pound small shrimp, peeled

¼ cup chopped fresh basil leaves

¼ cup diced red onions

1 teaspoon fine sea salt

1. Combine the lime juice, oil, and garlic in a large bowl. Add the shrimp, basil, onions, and salt. Stir well to combine.

2. Cover and refrigerate for 15 minutes before serving.

P/E ratio **4.0** • calories **339** • fat **11g** • protein **56g** • carbs **4g** • fiber **1g**

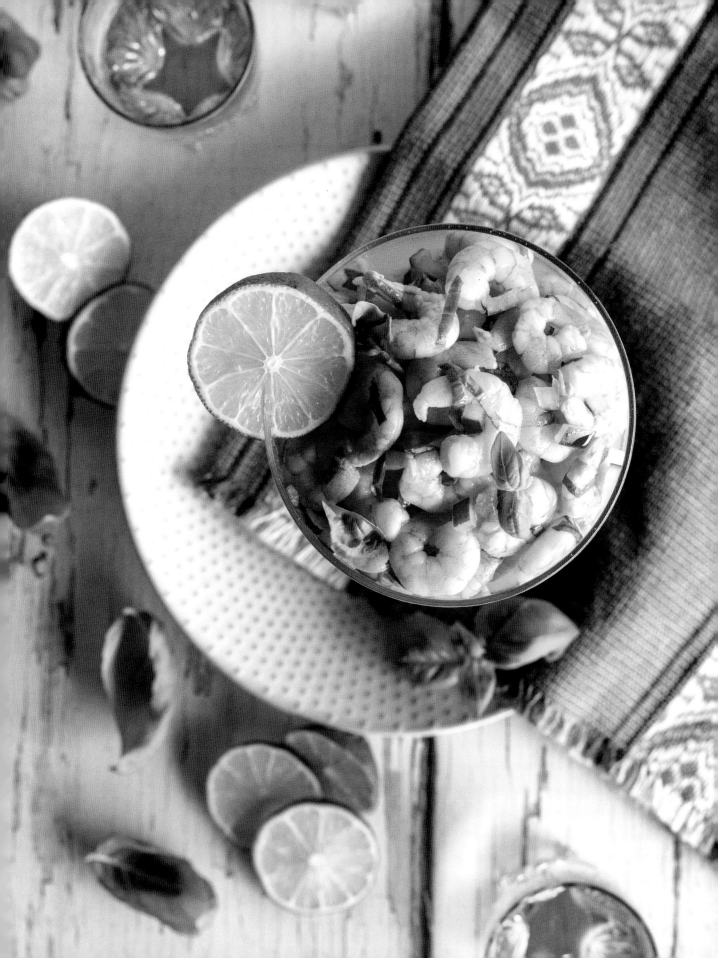

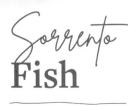

Sorrento Fish

     yield: 4 servings • prep time: 7 minutes • cook time: 22 minutes

When I was a teenager, I had a special family dinner at the famous chain restaurant Buca di Beppo in Minneapolis. I fell in love with one of their classic entrees, Salmon Sorrento, a delicate fish dish with the bright flavors of lemon, garlic, and capers. To this day, every time I recreate this dish at home, I'm reminded of the Italian music, the aroma of garlic, and the loud banter that drew me in the moment I entered the restaurant.

1 tablespoon coconut oil, lard, or tallow

3 cloves garlic, minced

¼ cup beef broth

¼ cup lemon juice

2 tablespoons capers, rinsed and drained

1 tablespoon tomato sauce

1 tablespoon chopped fresh parsley leaves, plus more for garnish

¼ teaspoon freshly ground black pepper

4 (6-ounce) cod fillets or other white fish fillets

2 teaspoons fine sea salt

1. Heat the oil in a large cast-iron skillet over medium-high heat. Add the garlic and sauté for 1 minute, until fragrant. Add the broth, lemon juice, capers, tomato sauce, parsley, and pepper. Cook, stirring often, until the liquid has reduced a bit, about 5 minutes.

2. While the sauce is simmering, rinse the cod fillets and pat dry with paper towels. Season on all sides with the salt.

3. Lower the heat under the skillet to medium. Use a rubber spatula to push the sauce to one side and place the cod in the skillet. Spoon the sauce over the fish. Cover the skillet and cook until the cod flakes easily with a fork, about 15 minutes.

4. Remove the fish from the skillet and place on a platter. Top with the sauce and garnish with more parsley.

P/E ratio **5.7** • calories **219** • fat **5g** • protein **40g** • carbs **3g** • fiber **1g**

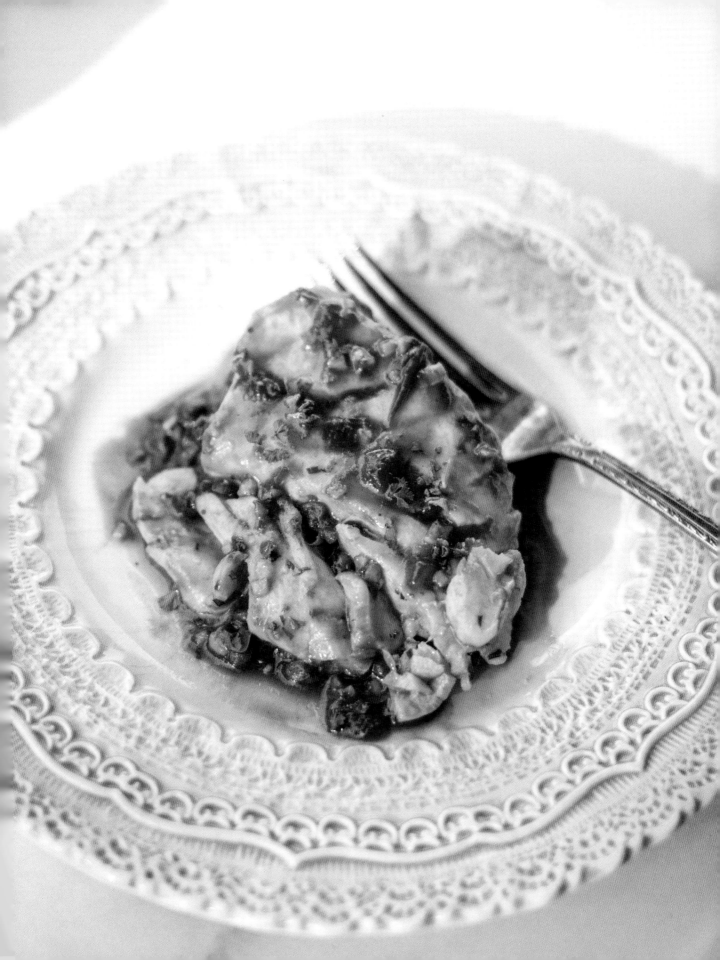

Peel-and-Eat
Ginger-Lime Shrimp

yield: 8 servings • prep time: 20 minutes • cook time: 5 minutes

Keeping the shells on keeps the shrimp juicy and succulent. To make this dish even easier to prepare, you can purchase shell-on extra-jumbo shrimp that have already been butterflied and deveined at your local seafood market.

2 pounds shell-on extra-jumbo shrimp, heads removed, deveined, and butterflied

2 tablespoons lime juice

2 teaspoons peeled and grated fresh ginger

1 teaspoon fine sea salt

Lime wedges, for serving (optional)

1. Place an oven rack 6 inches below the heating element (this usually means the second rack from the top of the oven). Turn the broiler to high (500°F).

2. Arrange the shrimp in a single layer on a rimmed baking sheet. In a small bowl, combine the lime juice, ginger, and salt, then drizzle over the shrimp.

3. Broil the shrimp until they are firm and the shells turn thoroughly pink, about 5 minutes.

4. Put the shrimp in a large serving bowl and place in the middle of the table along with lime wedges to squeeze over the shrimp, if desired. Enjoy immediately.

P/E ratio **11.7** • calories **269** • fat **4g** • protein **56g** • carbs **1g** • fiber **0.2g**

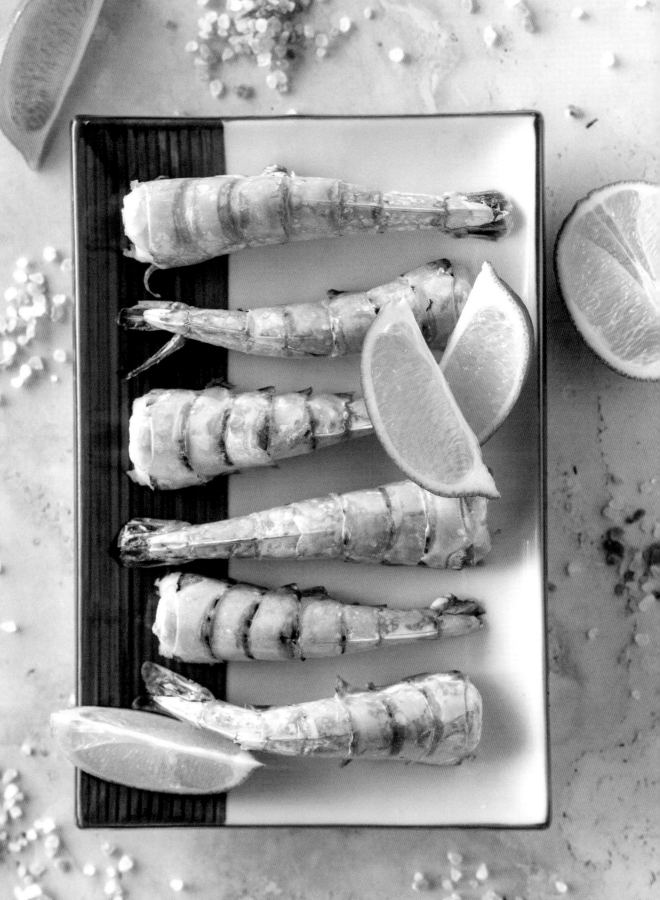

Halibut
with Ginger Sauce

    yield: 4 servings • prep time: 5 minutes • cook time: 23 minutes

1 cup beef or chicken broth

¼ cup diced yellow onions

2 cloves garlic, minced

¼ cup peeled and grated fresh ginger

2 tablespoons lime juice

1 teaspoon fish sauce

1 teaspoon fine sea salt

⅛ teaspoon liquid stevia, or more to taste

4 (4-ounce) halibut fillets

Cilantro leaves, for garnish (optional)

Lime wedges, for serving (optional)

1. Put the broth in a medium-sized saucepan and bring to a gentle boil over medium-high heat. Add the onions, garlic, ginger, lime juice, fish sauce, salt, and stevia; lower the heat to a simmer and cook until the onions are soft and the liquid has reduced a bit, 15 to 30 minutes.

2. Blend with an immersion blender into a smooth puree. Taste and add more stevia if desired.

3. Add the halibut fillets to the sauce and cook until the fish flakes easily with a fork, about 7 minutes. Remove the pan from the heat.

4. Place a fillet in each bowl and top with the sauce. If desired, garnish with cilantro leaves and serve with lime wedges.

P/E ratio **4.9** • calories **292** • fat **6g** • protein **49g** • carbs **5g** • fiber **1g**

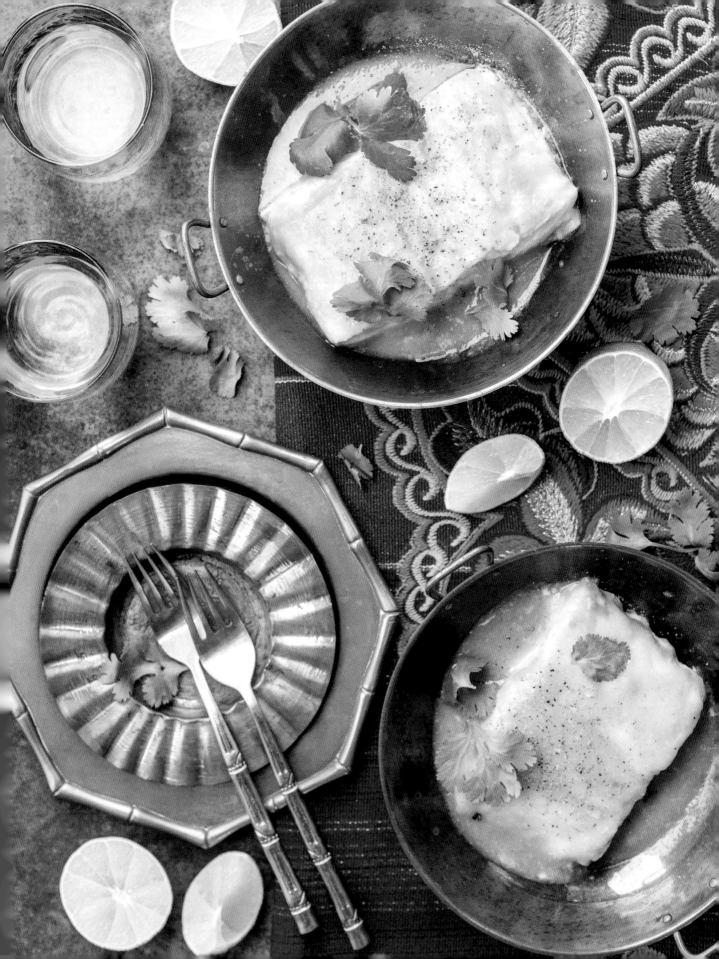

Baked Garlic
and Herb Lobster Tails

   yield: 4 servings • prep time: 5 minutes • cook time: 5 minutes

8 (8-ounce) lobster tails

2 tablespoons lemon juice

3 cloves garlic, minced

¾ teaspoon fine sea salt

½ teaspoon smoked paprika

½ teaspoon dried parsley

½ teaspoon dried thyme leaves

1. Place an oven rack 6 inches below the heating element (usually this means the second rack from the top of the oven). Turn the broiler to high (500°F).

2. Use kitchen shears to cut the tops of the lobster shells lengthwise down the middle. Pull the shells apart a little to expose the meat. Place the lobster tails on a rimmed baking sheet.

3. In a small bowl, stir together the lemon juice, garlic, salt, paprika, parsley, and thyme. Brush the mixture evenly on the lobster tails, making sure the seasoning gets into the meat.

4. Broil until the lobster meat becomes firm and opaque or the internal temperature reaches 140°F. Serve warm.

P/E ratio **13.0** • calories **415** • fat **5g** • protein **86g** • carbs **2g** • fiber **0.4g**

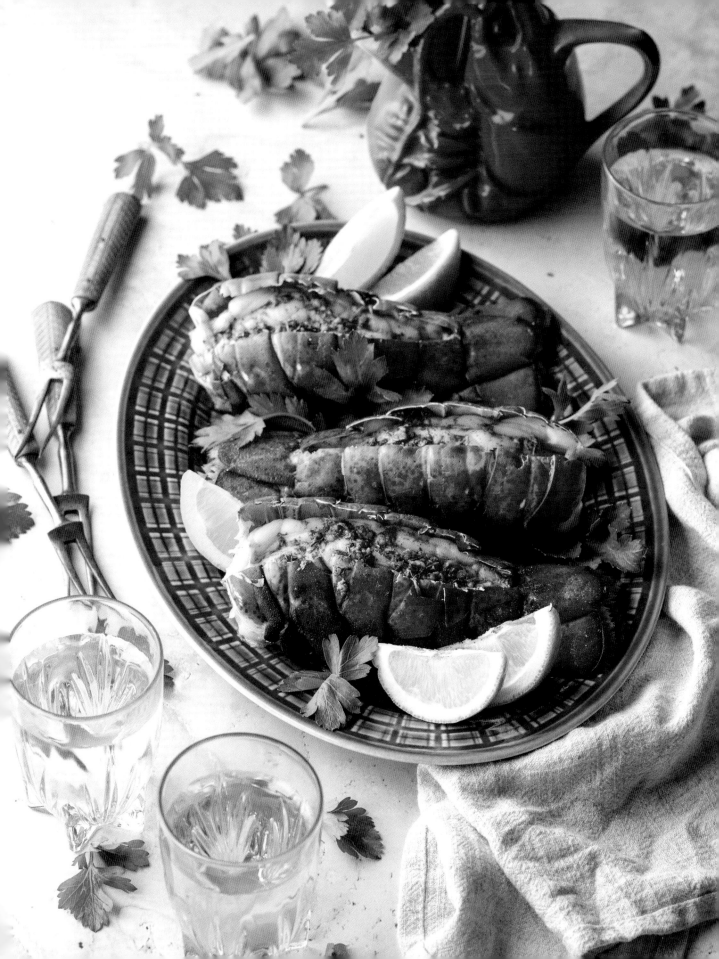

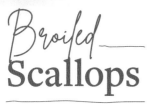

Broiled Scallops

    yield: 2 servings • prep time: 4 minutes • cook time: 4 minutes

12 medium-sized sea scallops

Duck fat spray or coconut oil spray, for greasing

1 teaspoon garlic salt or fine sea salt

¾ teaspoon freshly ground black pepper

Fresh parsley leaves, for garnish (optional)

1. Place an oven rack 6 inches below the heating element (usually this means the second rack from the top of the oven). Turn the broiler to high (500°F). Line a rimmed baking sheet with parchment paper.

2. Rinse the scallops and pat completely dry. Arrange them on the prepared baking sheet. Spray the scallops with duck fat spray and season on all sides with the garlic salt and pepper.

3. Broil until the scallops are firm and opaque, 6 to 10 minutes. Garnish with parsley, if desired. Serve warm.

P/E ratio **3.4** • calories **240** • fat **5g** • protein **40g** • carbs **7g** • fiber **0.4g**

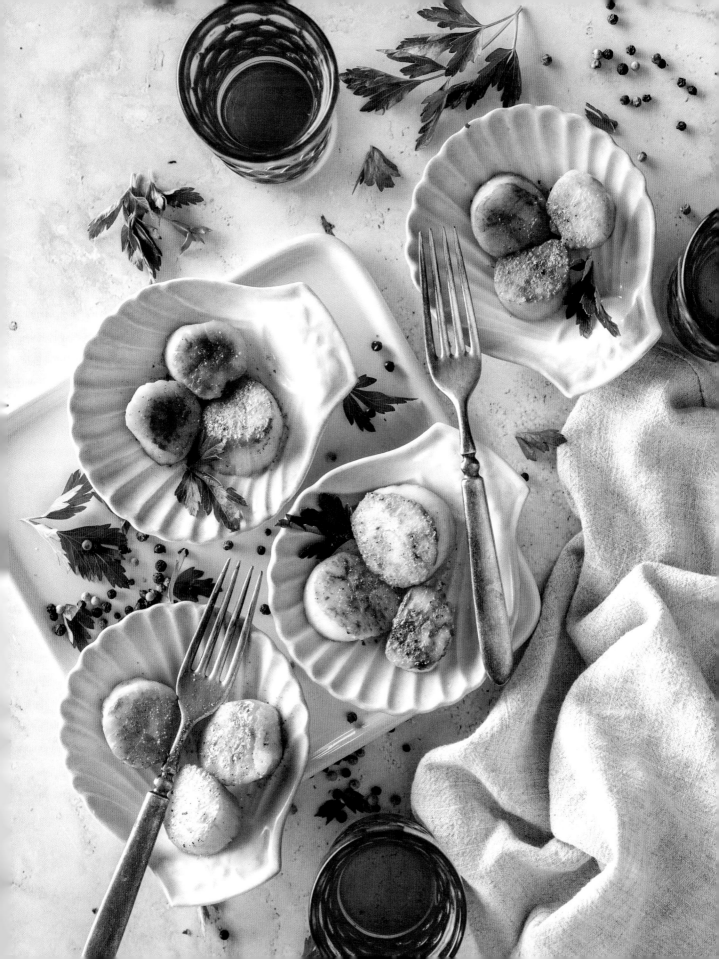

Mediterranean-Style
Grilled Swordfish

   yield: 2 servings • prep time: 5 minutes, plus 15 minutes to marinate • cook time: 12 minutes

This easy recipe showcases fresh fish and a delicious marinade with the Mediterranean flavors of cumin, garlic, and more. It's quick, too—just a few minutes of marinating while the grill is heating.

6 cloves garlic, peeled

⅓ cup fish stock or beef broth

2 tablespoons lemon juice

1 teaspoon ground coriander

¾ teaspoon ground cumin

1 teaspoon smoked paprika

1 teaspoon fine sea salt

½ teaspoon freshly ground black pepper

2 (8-ounce) swordfish fillets

Duck fat or coconut oil, for greasing

Fresh parsley leaves, for garnish (optional)

Lemon wedges, for serving (optional)

1. Make the marinade: In a food processor, blend the garlic, broth, lemon juice, coriander, cumin, paprika, salt, and pepper until smooth.

2. Place the swordfish fillets in a shallow dish and apply the marinade generously on both sides. Set the fish aside to marinate for about 15 minutes while you prepare the grill.

3. Lightly grease the grates of a grill with duck fat. Heat the grill to high heat.

4. Remove the fish from the marinade, shake off the excess moisture, and place them on the part of the grill that isn't directly above the flame. Cook the fish on both sides until it is firm and opaque and flakes easily with a fork, about 6 minutes per side.

5. Transfer the fish to serving plates. If desired, garnish with parsley and serve with lemon wedges.

P/E ratio **3.6** • calories **364** • fat **12g** • protein **58g** • carbs **5g** • fiber **1g**

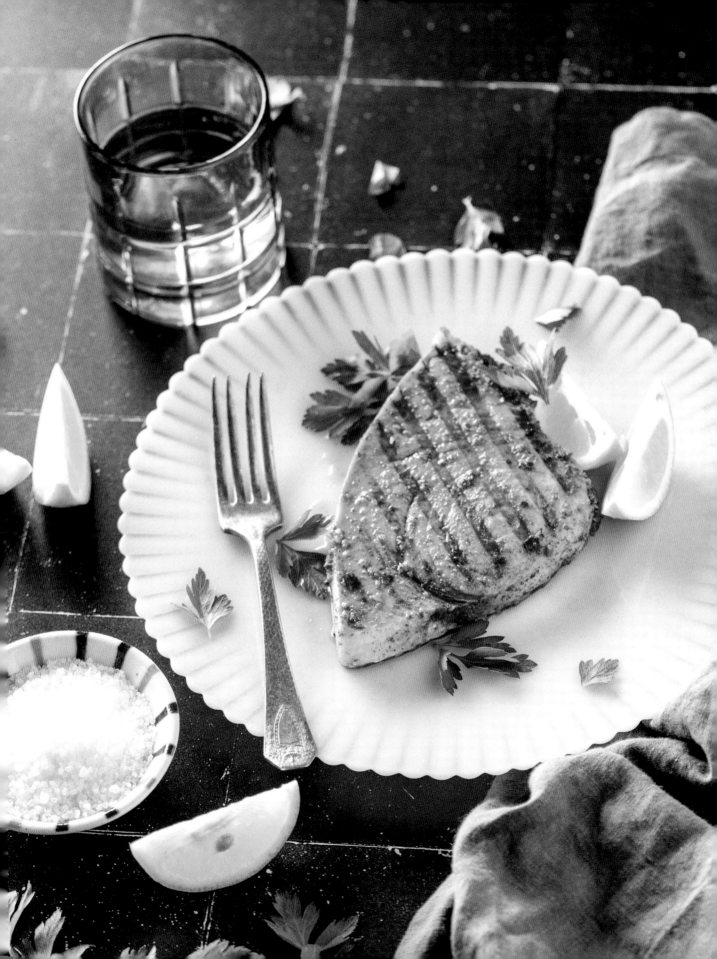

Shrimp
Scampi

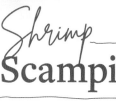

yield: 4 servings • prep time: 5 minutes • cook time: 6 minutes

2 tablespoons extra-virgin olive oil

2 tablespoons seafood stock or chicken broth

1 tablespoon lemon juice

2 cloves garlic, minced

2 tablespoons chopped fresh basil leaves, plus whole leaves for garnish

1 teaspoon fine sea salt

1 pound large shrimp, peeled and deveined

1. Preheat the oven to 350°F.

2. Combine the oil, stock, lemon juice, garlic, basil, and salt in a small casserole dish. Add the shrimp and mix well. Bake until the shrimp are firm and opaque, 6 to 8 minutes.

3. Garnish with basil leaves and serve.

P/E ratio **2.8** • calories **197** • fat **9g** • protein **28g** • carbs **1g** • fiber **0.1g**

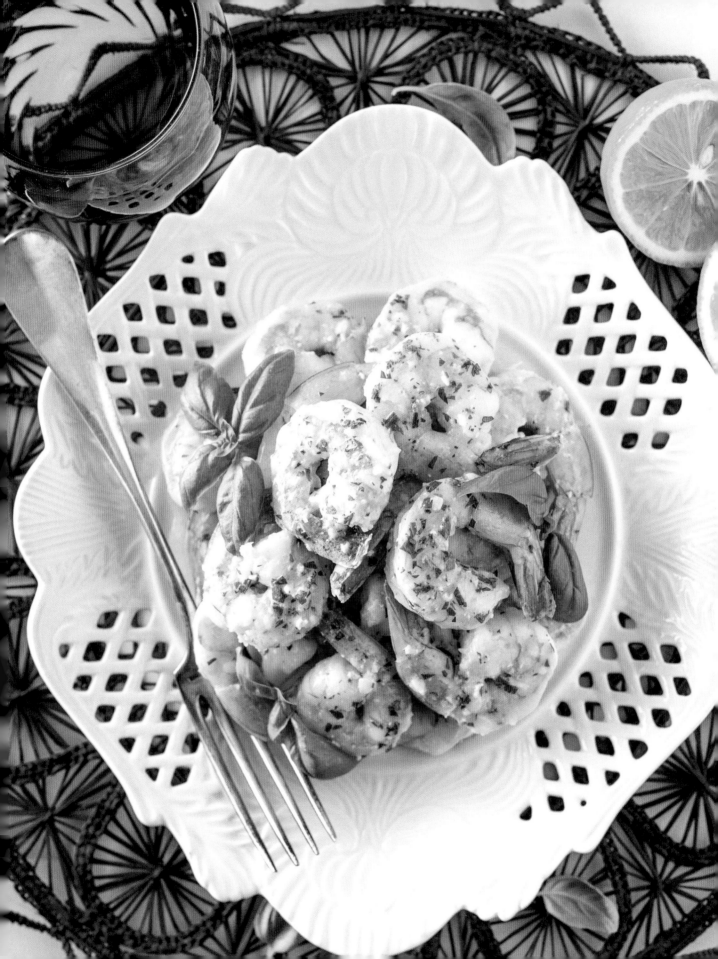

Salmon in
Ramen Broth

   yield: 4 servings • prep time: 5 minutes • cook time: 20 minutes

If you love ramen, you are going to love this filling salmon meal! The delicious broth is simple to make yet so flavorful.

1 tablespoon coconut oil, lard, or tallow

1 tablespoon toasted sesame oil

4 (3-ounce) skinless salmon fillets

Fine sea salt

Freshly ground black pepper

½ cup minced onions

2 cloves garlic, minced

1 tablespoon red pepper flakes, or 1½ teaspoons cayenne pepper

1 quart chicken broth

2 tablespoons wheat-free tamari

1 tablespoon coconut vinegar or unseasoned rice vinegar

1 tablespoon peeled and grated fresh ginger

1 tablespoon tomato paste

Thinly sliced green onions, for garnish

1. Heat the oils in a large saucepan over medium heat. Pat the salmon fillets dry and season on all sides with a pinch each of salt and pepper. Place the salmon in the hot oil and cook on both sides until they are firm and opaque and flake easily with a fork, about 4 minutes per side.

2. Remove the salmon fillets from the saucepan with a slotted spoon and place in four serving bowls, leaving the fat in the pan and keeping the pan on the heat. Turn the heat down to low.

3. Add the onions, garlic, and red pepper flakes and cook until the onions are translucent, about 4 minutes.

4. Increase the heat to medium-high. Add the chicken broth, tamari, vinegar, ginger, and tomato paste and bring to a simmer. Simmer for 8 minutes, then taste and add more salt and pepper as needed.

5. Ladle the broth over the fish. Garnish with green onions.

P/E ratio **2.5** • calories **330** • fat **14g** • protein **45g** • carbs **5g** • fiber **1g**

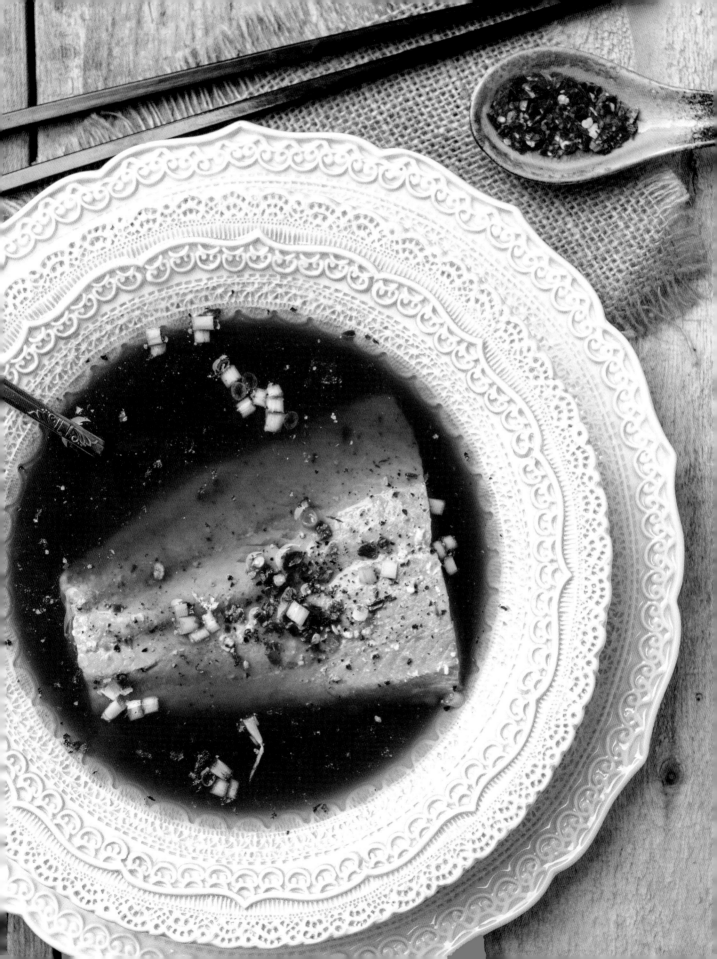

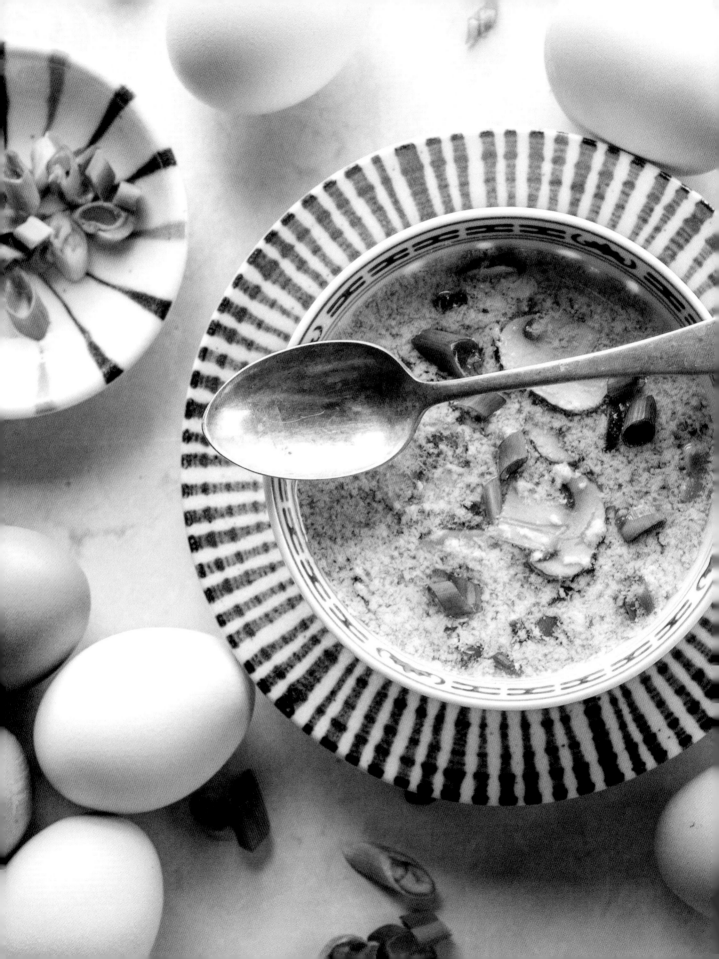

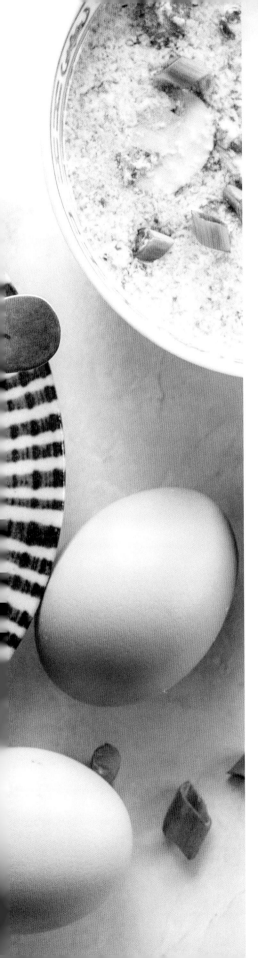

chapter 3
Sides & Snacks

Egg Drop Soup / 210

Chicken Soup / 212

Meatball Soup / 214

Egg Salad Sandwiches / 216

Turkey Sandwich / 218

Cool Ranch Chips and Dip / 220

Venison Jerky / 222

Salmon Jerky / 224

Fried "Rice" / 226

Thanksgiving Stuffing / 228

Egg
Drop Soup

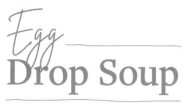 yield: 2 servings • prep time: 5 minutes • cook time: 5 minutes

1 quart chicken broth

6 ounces button mushrooms, thinly sliced

3 green onions, thinly sliced, plus more for garnish if desired

3 tablespoons wheat-free tamari

2 teaspoons peeled and grated fresh ginger

1 teaspoon fish sauce, or ½ teaspoon fine sea salt

¼ teaspoon freshly ground black pepper

8 large egg whites, or 1 cup 100% liquid egg whites, lightly beaten

1. Put the broth, mushrooms, green onions, tamari, ginger, fish sauce, and pepper in a large saucepan and bring to a boil over medium-high heat. Lower the heat to a simmer and cook until the mushrooms have softened, about 3 minutes.

2. Reduce the heat to low. Slowly pour in the egg whites while stirring. The eggs will form ribbons and cook in about 2 minutes.

3. Divide the soup between two bowls. Garnish with more green onions, if desired, and serve warm.

P/E ratio **4.6** • calories **218** • fat **3g** • protein **41g** • carbs **8g** • fiber **2g**

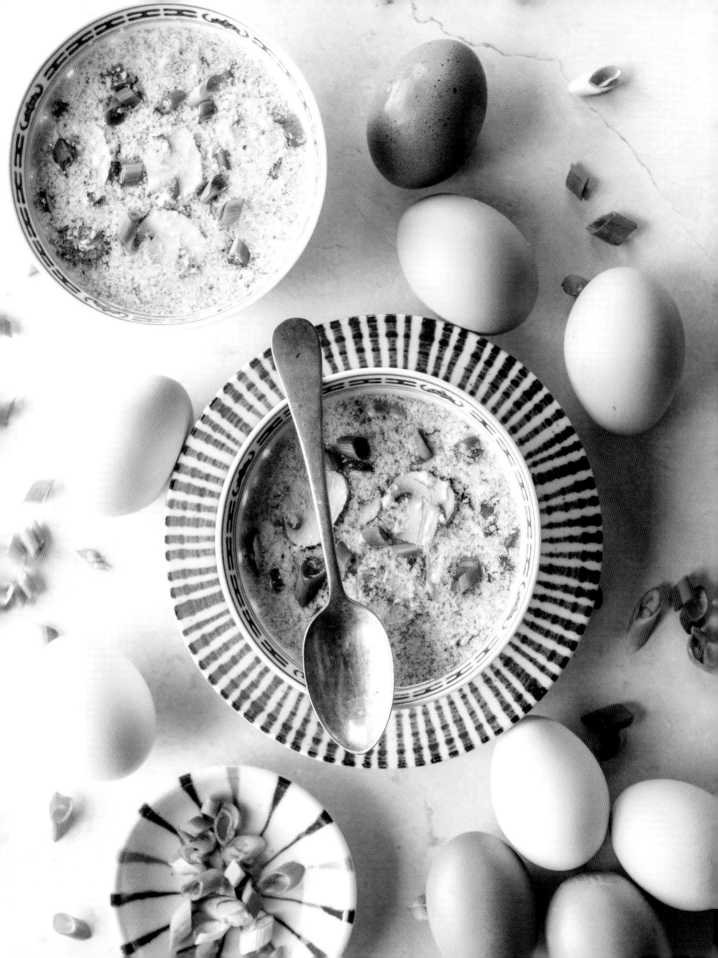

Chicken Soup

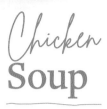

yield: 4 servings • prep time: 8 minutes • cook time: 13 minutes

1 tablespoon coconut oil, lard, or tallow

¼ cup diced yellow onions

2 cloves garlic, finely minced

18 ounces boneless, skinless chicken breasts, cut into 1-inch cubes

2 quarts chicken broth

Fine sea salt

Freshly ground black pepper

Chopped fresh herbs, such as thyme, parsley, or cilantro, for garnish (optional)

1. Heat the oil in a large saucepan over medium heat. Add the onions and garlic and sauté until the onions are translucent, about 5 minutes.

2. Add the chicken to the pan and sauté until the chicken is firm and opaque, about 5 minutes. Pour in the broth and bring to a simmer for 3 minutes. Season to taste with salt and pepper.

3. Garnish with herbs, if desired, and serve hot.

P/E ratio **3.5** • calories **386** • fat **15g** • protein **58g** • carbs **2g** • fiber **0.3g**

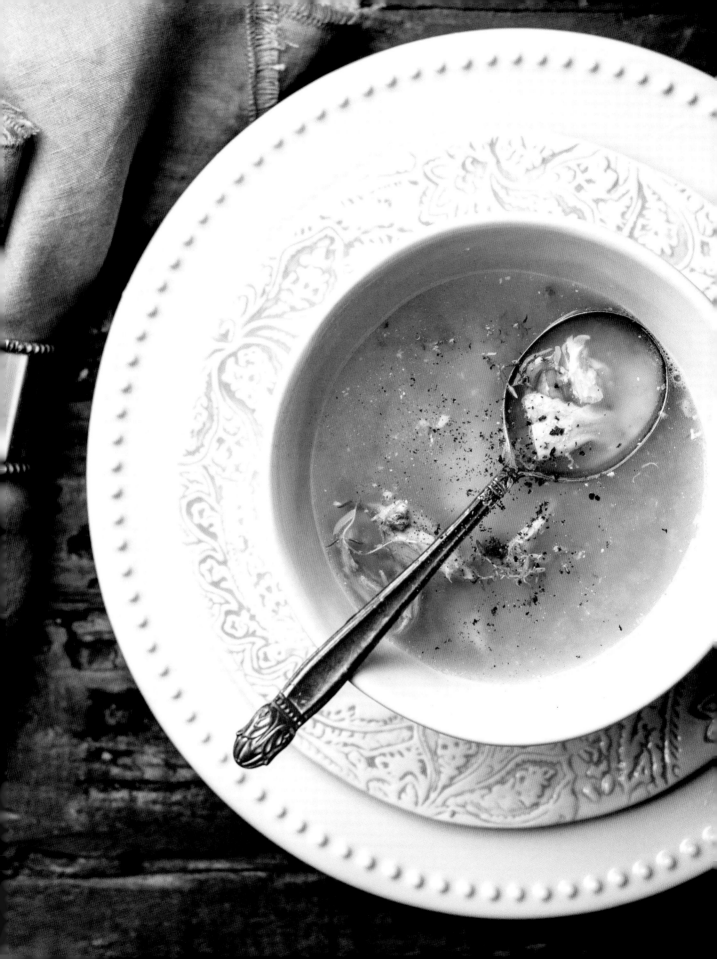

Meatball Soup

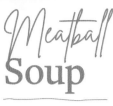

yield: 8 servings • prep time: 8 minutes • cook time: 15 minutes

Meatballs:

2 pounds 95% lean ground beef

¼ cup chopped yellow onions

1 clove garlic, minced

2 tablespoons beef broth or water

1½ teaspoons dried thyme leaves

2 large egg whites

1 teaspoon fine sea salt

1 teaspoon fish sauce (optional)

Broth:

1 quart beef broth

¼ cup diced yellow onions

1 teaspoon dried thyme leaves

Fine sea salt

Fresh thyme sprigs, for garnish (optional)

1. Preheat the oven to 400°F. Line a rimmed baking sheet with parchment paper.

2. Put the ground beef, onions, garlic, broth, thyme, egg whites, salt, and fish sauce, if using, in a large bowl and mix the ingredients with your hands until well combined.

3. Shape the meat mixture into 1¼-inch balls and place on the prepared baking sheet. Bake until golden brown and no longer pink inside, about 15 minutes.

4. Meanwhile, prepare the onion broth: In a large saucepan, combine the broth, onions, and thyme and bring to a boil over medium-high heat. Cook, uncovered, until the onions are very soft, about 10 minutes. Taste and add salt if needed.

5. Ladle the broth into serving bowls and divide the meatballs evenly among the bowls. Garnish with thyme sprigs, if desired, and serve hot.

P/E ratio **3.9** • calories **218** • fat **8g** • protein **34g** • carbs **1g** • fiber **0.3g**

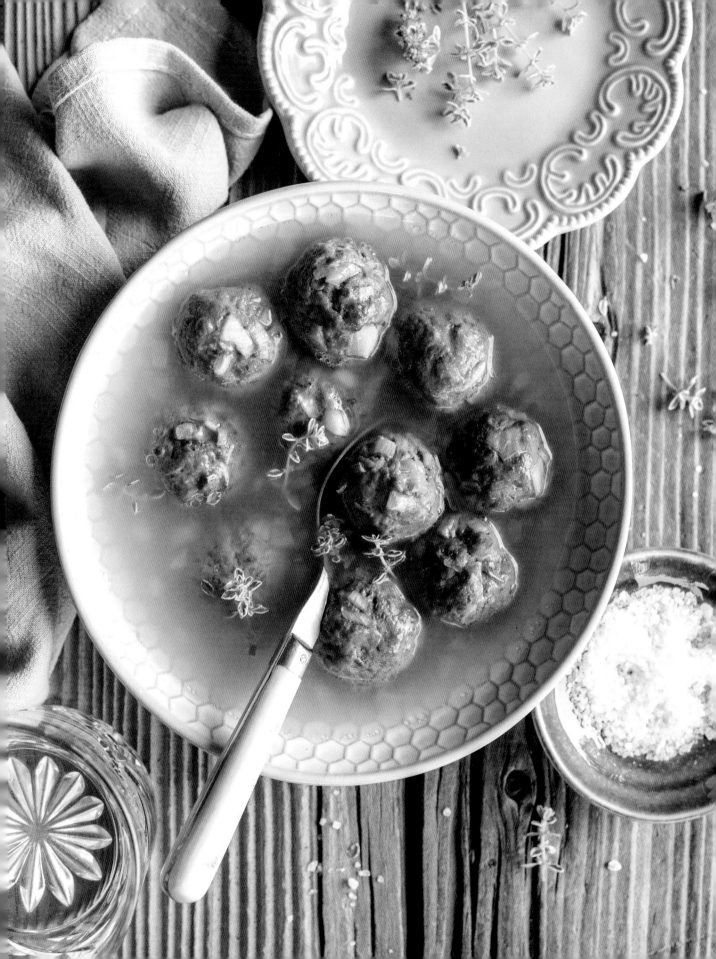

Egg Salad Sandwiches

  yield: 6 sandwiches (1 per serving) • prep time: 10 minutes • cook time: 8 minutes

Buns:

Duck fat spray or coconut oil spray, for greasing

3 large egg whites

2 tablespoons unflavored egg white protein powder

Egg Salad:

8 large hard-boiled egg whites

2 large hard-boiled egg yolks

¼ cup Dijon or prepared yellow mustard

1 tablespoon chopped fresh dill, or 1 teaspoon dried dill weed

½ teaspoon fine sea salt

¼ teaspoon freshly ground black pepper

1. Preheat the oven to 375°F. Lightly grease a rimmed baking sheet with duck fat spray.

2. Make the buns: Put the egg whites in a large, grease-free bowl and beat with an electric handheld mixer on high speed until stiff peaks form. Fold in the protein powder; the batter will be stiff. Form into 12 balls, each about 2 inches across, and arrange on the prepared baking sheet. Bake for 5 minutes, then turn off the oven, keep the oven door shut, and leave the buns in the oven for about 3 minutes more.

3. Meanwhile, make the egg salad: Chop the egg whites into small pieces and put in a large bowl. Add the egg yolks, mustard, dill, salt, and pepper; mash well with a fork. Taste and add more salt and pepper if needed.

4. To assemble the sandwiches, divide the egg salad into 6 equal portions and spread each portion on the bottom of a bun. Close with another bun to form a sandwich. Serve immediately.

P/E ratio **2.8** • calories **136** • fat **5g** • protein **19g** • carbs **2g** • fiber **0.1g**

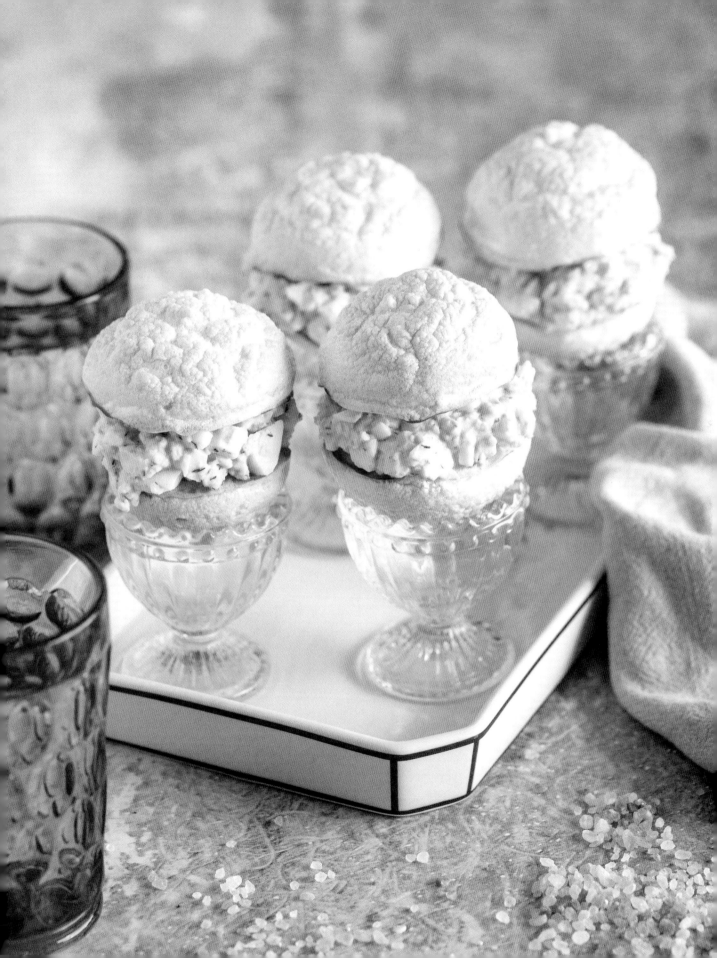

Turkey
Sandwich

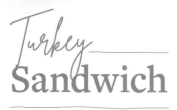

  yield: 1 serving • prep time: 5 minutes (not including time to make bread)

2 slices Protein-Sparing Bread (page 270)

4 ounces thinly sliced deli turkey breast

2 tablespoons Dijon or prepared yellow mustard

1. Place a slice of bread on a plate. Top with the turkey.

2. Spread the mustard on the other slice of bread and place on top of the turkey to close the sandwich. Serve immediately.

P/E ratio **12.0** • calories **258** • fat **3g** • protein **48g** • carbs **1g** • fiber **0g**

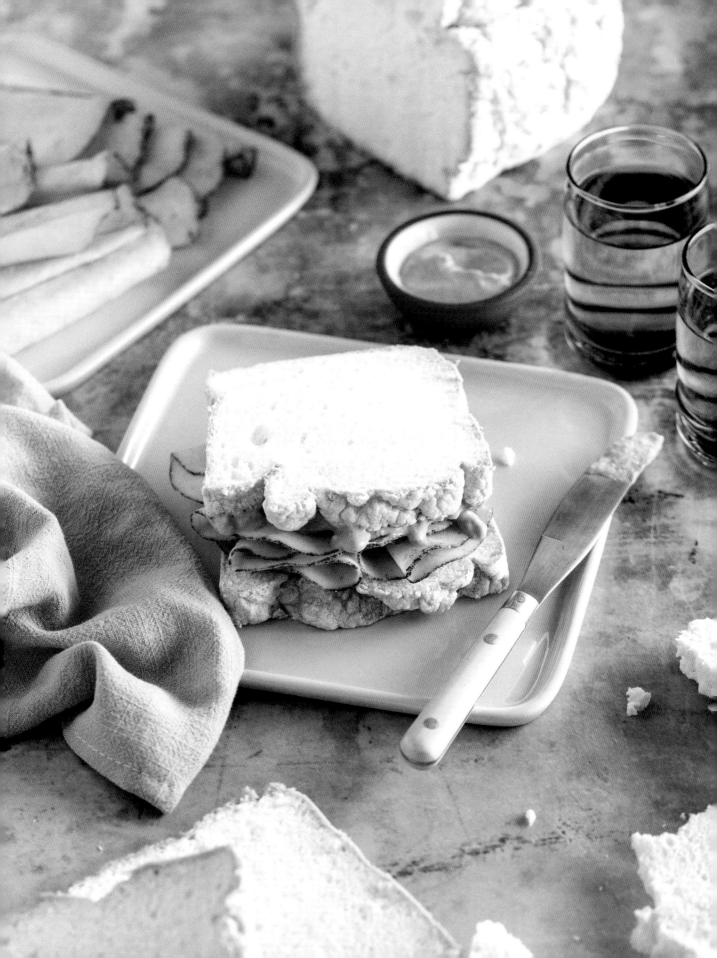

Cool Ranch Chips and Dip

  yield: 4 servings (with dip left over) • prep time: 10 minutes • cook time: 8 to 10 hours

This ranch dip got a two thumbs-up from one of my recipe testers! I also love it smeared on my Protein-Sparing Bread (page 270).

Chips:

8 ounces thin round slices deli chicken, turkey, or ham

2 teaspoons dried parsley

2 teaspoons garlic powder

2 teaspoons onion powder

2 teaspoons smoked paprika

1½ teaspoons dried dill weed

1 teaspoon dried chives

Dip (*makes 1½ cups, 2 tablespoons per serving*):

6 large hard-boiled egg whites, or ¾ cup 100% liquid egg whites, lightly scrambled

⅓ cup beef broth

1 teaspoon apple cider vinegar or lemon juice

1 tablespoon dried parsley

1½ teaspoons garlic powder

1½ teaspoons onion powder

¾ teaspoon dried dill weed

¾ teaspoon fine sea salt

½ teaspoon dried chives

1. Make the chips: Preheat the oven to 145°F. Line 3 rimmed baking sheets with parchment paper.

2. Arrange the deli meat on the parchment paper in a single layer.

3. In a small bowl, stir together the parsley, garlic powder, onion powder, paprika, dill weed, and chives until well combined. Sprinkle the deli meat with the seasoning mix.

4. Place the baking sheets in the oven to dehydrate the meat slices until crispy, 8 to 10 hours. Let cool completely before serving.

5. Make the dip: Put all of the ingredients in a wide-mouth jar and use an immersion blender to puree until completely smooth, scraping down the sides as needed with a small rubber spatula.

6. Serve the chips with the dip. Store leftover chips in an airtight container for up to 10 days and leftover dip in a jar in the refrigerator for up to a week.

Chips:
P/E ratio **11.0** • calories **61** • fat **1g** • protein **11g** • carbs **1g** • fiber **1g**

Dip:
P/E ratio **4.0** • calories **11** • fat **0.1g** • protein **2g** • carbs **0.5g** • fiber **0.1g**

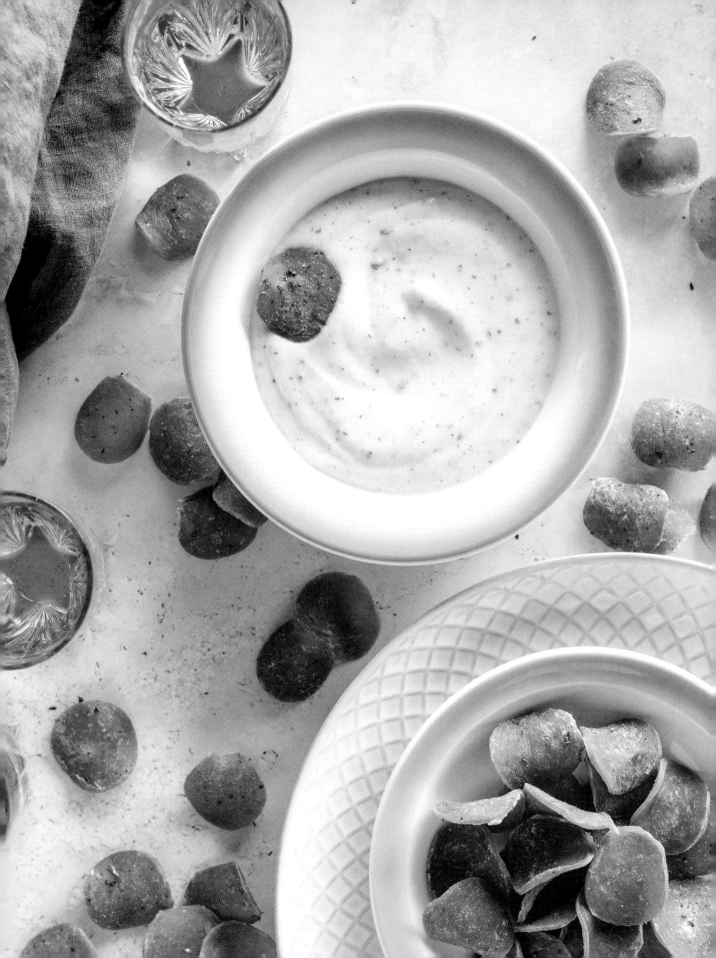

Venison
Jerky

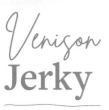

yield: 8 servings • prep time: 5 minutes, plus 3 hours to freeze and marinate • cook time: 1 hour 15 minutes or 6 hours, depending on method

Not only is jerky a delicious snack, but it's also the ultimate portable food. We often pack it on camping trips. However, it's hard to find store-bought jerky that doesn't contain gluten or sugar. Thankfully, jerky is extremely easy to make, and you can use a dehydrator, a smoker, or the oven. I like to make a double batch and store it in the freezer.

You can use any type of smoker you have to prepare this jerky, as long as it allows you to perfume the meat with wood smoke. Follow the manufacturer's instructions for how to use wood chips, if applicable. If you use a pellet smoker, you get a smoky scent from the pellets, so you don't need wood chips.

1 pound boneless venison or beef tenderloin

½ cup wheat-free tamari

2 tablespoons lime juice

1 tablespoon MCT oil or macadamia nut oil

¼ teaspoon liquid stevia

1 tablespoon peeled and grated fresh ginger

1 teaspoon minced garlic

1 teaspoon fine sea salt

Special Equipment (optional):

Food dehydrator or smoker

1. Place the meat in the freezer for 1 hour to make it easier to slice cleanly. Cut the meat across the grain into strips, about 1 inch wide and ⅛ inch thick.

2. Combine the tamari, lime juice, oil, stevia, ginger, and garlic in a large shallow bowl. Submerge the meat strips in the marinade, cover, and refrigerate for at least 2 hours or overnight.

3. Remove the meat from the marinade and sprinkle with the salt.

4. *If using a dehydrator,* place the meat strips in the dehydrator, not touching each other, and set the dehydrator to 170°F.

   If using the oven, preheat the oven to 160°F. Place a rimmed baking sheet on the bottom of the oven (or bottom rack) to catch drips. Arrange the meat strips directly on the middle rack, not touching each other. (Alternatively, place a wire rack on a rimmed baking sheet and arrange the strips on the rack.)

   Dehydrate the meat until it has dried to the desired chewiness, 6 to 8 hours. (For a chewier jerky, dehydrate for less time.)

   If using a smoker, preheat the smoker to 160°F. Arrange the meat strips on the smoker grates and smoke for 30 minutes. Increase the temperature to 230°F and continue to smoke for 45 minutes to 1 hour longer, until it has reached the desired chewiness.

5. Let cool completely before serving. Store the jerky in an airtight container in the refrigerator for up to 10 days. If you vacuum-seal it, it will keep for up to 3 weeks.

P/E ratio **3.8** • calories **114** • fat **3g** • protein **19g** • carbs **2g** • fiber **0g**

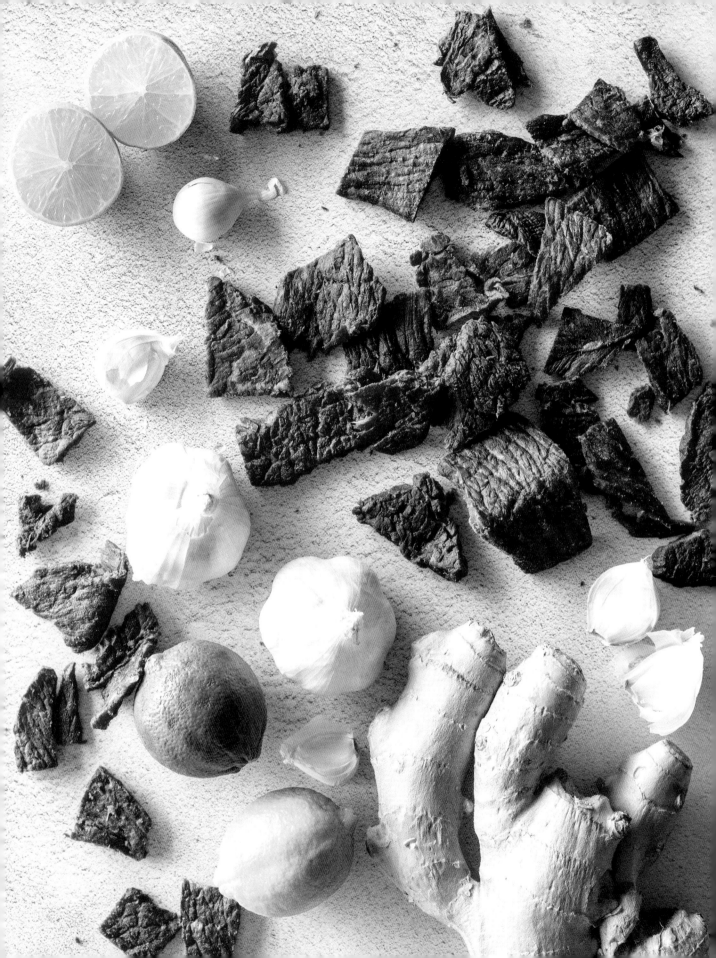

Salmon
Jerky

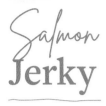

   yield: 8 servings • prep time: 10 minutes, plus 2 hours to marinate • cook time: 3 hours

1 (1¼-pound) skinless salmon fillet, pin bones removed

½ cup wheat-free tamari

2 teaspoons lime juice

1 tablespoon peeled and grated fresh ginger

1 teaspoon minced garlic

⅛ teaspoon liquid stevia

1. Cut the salmon into strips, about ¼ inch thick and 4 inches long.

2. Combine the remaining ingredients in a large shallow bowl. Submerge the salmon strips in the marinade, cover, and refrigerate for at least 2 hours or up to overnight.

3. Preheat the oven to 145°F. Line three baking sheets with parchment paper.

4. Remove the salmon strips from the marinade and arrange them on the prepared baking sheets. Put in the oven to dehydrate until completely dry to the touch yet still pliable, about 3 hours, turning the strips over halfway through. Remove the jerky from the oven and let it cool completely before serving.

5. Store the jerky in an airtight container in the refrigerator for up to 10 days. If you vacuum-seal it, it will keep for up to 3 weeks.

P/E ratio **2.5** • calories **28** • fat **1g** • protein **5g** • carbs **1g** • fiber **0g**

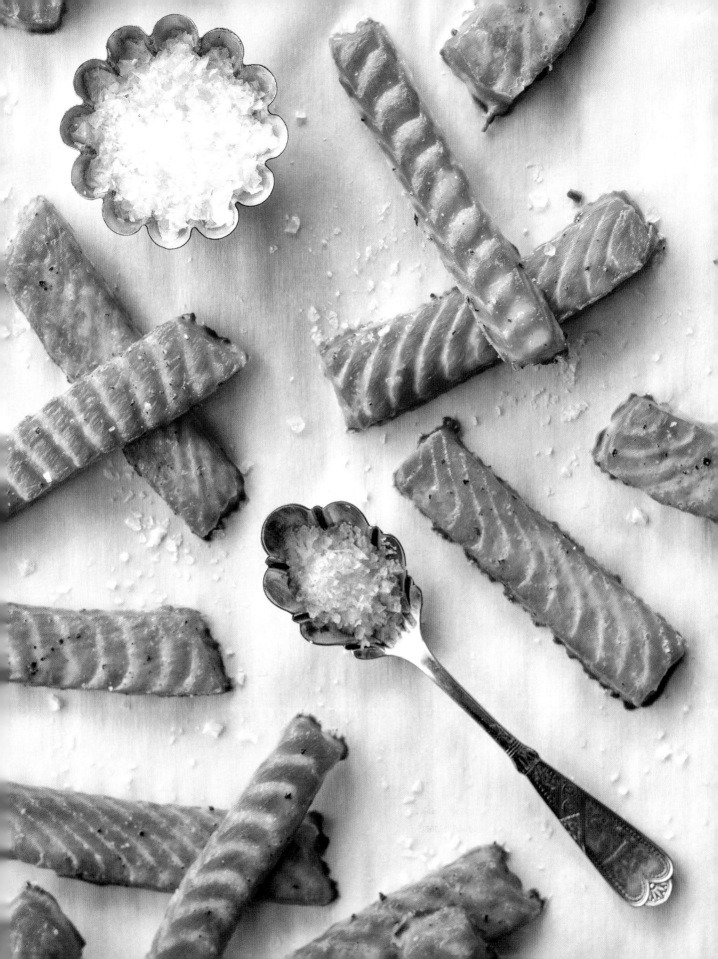

Fried "Rice"

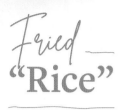

  yield: 4 servings • prep time: 5 minutes • cook time: 9 minutes

12 large egg whites

2 tablespoons beef broth

1 teaspoon wheat-free tamari

1 teaspoon coconut oil, lard, or tallow

¼ cup diced yellow onions

1 clove garlic, minced

For Garnish (optional):

Red pepper flakes

Thinly sliced green onions

1. Put the egg whites, broth, and tamari in a large bowl and whisk until well combined.

2. Heat the oil in a large nonstick skillet over medium heat. Add the onions and garlic and sauté until the onions are translucent, about 2 minutes. Pour the egg white mixture into the skillet and cook, whisking and scraping the bottom of the pan, until the mixture thickens and small curds form, about 7 minutes.

3. Transfer the fried "rice" to a serving platter. Garnish with red pepper flakes and/or green onions, if desired, and serve. *Note:* The fried "rice" tends to release moisture upon standing. Simply sop it up with paper towels before serving.

P/E ratio **5.2** • calories **59** • fat **0.3g** • protein **11g** • carbs **2g** • fiber **0.2g**

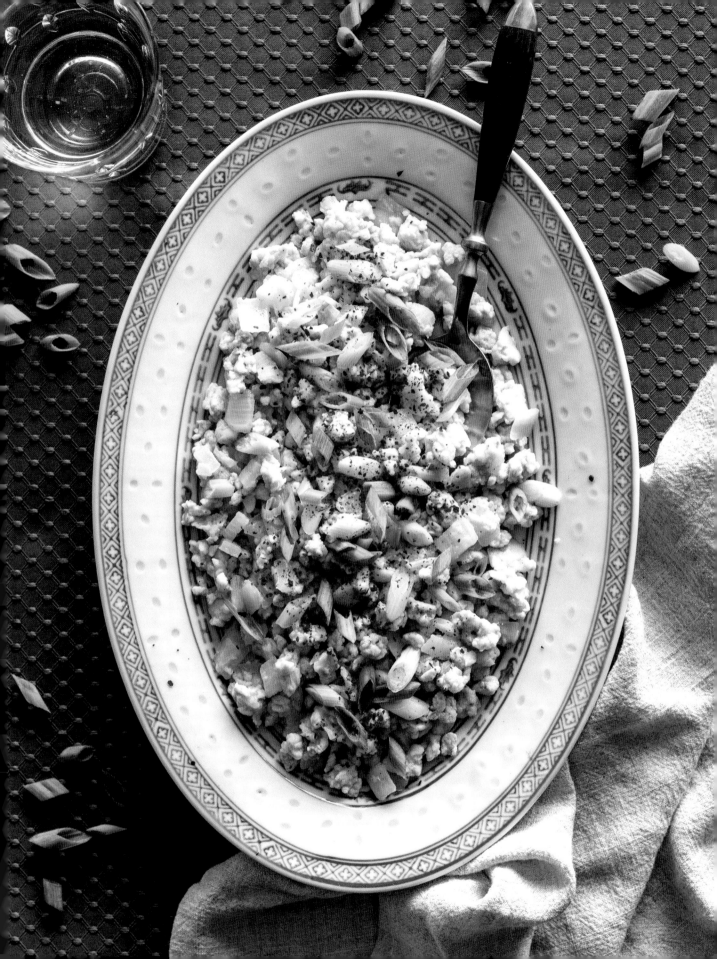

Thanksgiving Stuffing

  yield: 12 servings • prep time: 5 minutes (not including time to make bread) • cook time: 50 minutes

Duck fat spray or coconut oil spray, for greasing

1 tablespoon coconut oil, lard, or tallow

8 ounces button mushrooms, thinly sliced

2 stalks celery, chopped

¼ cup chopped yellow onions

1 pound 95% lean ground turkey

1 teaspoon dried rubbed sage

1 teaspoon poultry seasoning

1 loaf Protein-Sparing Bread (page 270), cut into ⅓-inch cubes

1 cup chicken broth

1 teaspoon fine sea salt

½ teaspoon freshly ground black pepper

4 large egg whites, lightly beaten

Fresh sage leaves, for garnish (optional)

Chopped fresh parsley leaves, for garnish (optional)

1. Preheat the oven to 325°F. Lightly grease a 1½- to 2-quart casserole dish with duck fat spray.

2. Heat the oil in a large cast-iron skillet over medium heat. Add the mushrooms, celery, and onions and sauté until the vegetables are tender, about 4 minutes.

3. Add the ground turkey, sage, and poultry seasoning and sauté, cook up the turkey into small pieces with a spatula, until no pink remains, about 4 minutes. Remove the pan from the heat.

4. Arrange the bread cubes in the prepared casserole dish. Add the turkey and vegetable mixture, broth, salt, pepper, and egg whites and mix well. Cover the dish with foil and bake for 40 minutes. Remove the foil and bake until the top is golden brown, 5 to 10 minutes more.

5. Garnish with sage and parsley, if desired. Serve warm.

P/E ratio **5.3** • calories **106** • fat **2g** • protein **19g** • carbs **2g** • fiber **0.4g**

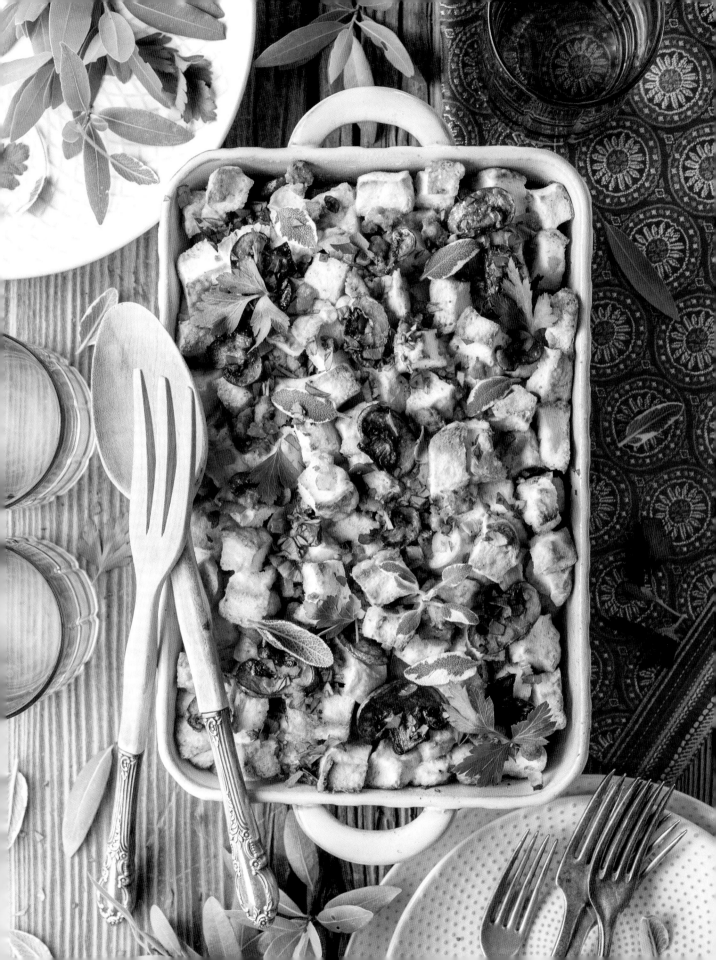

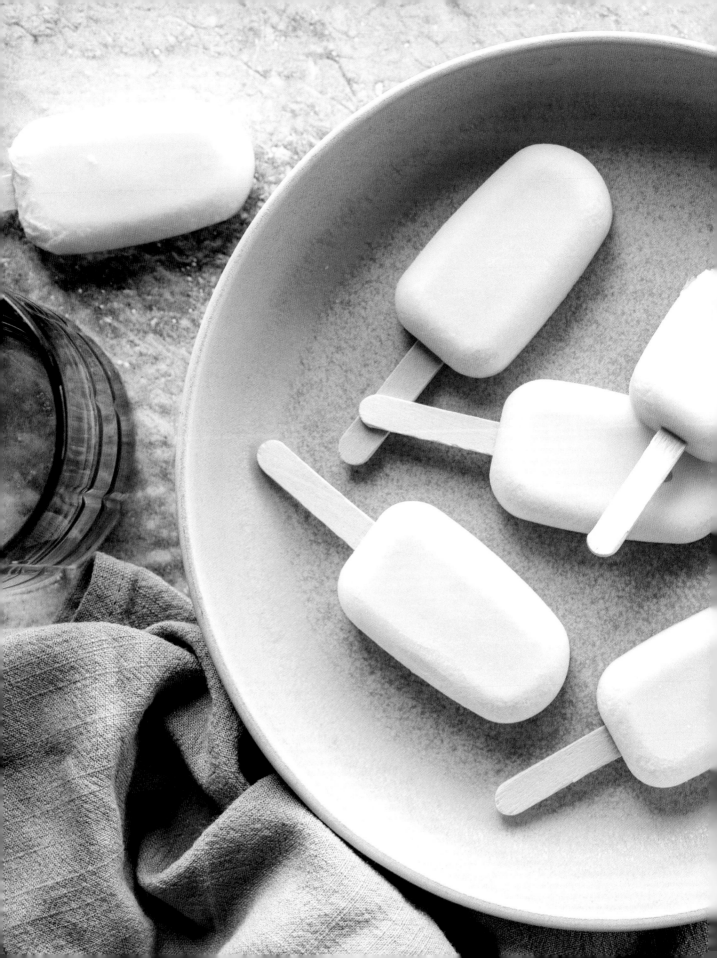

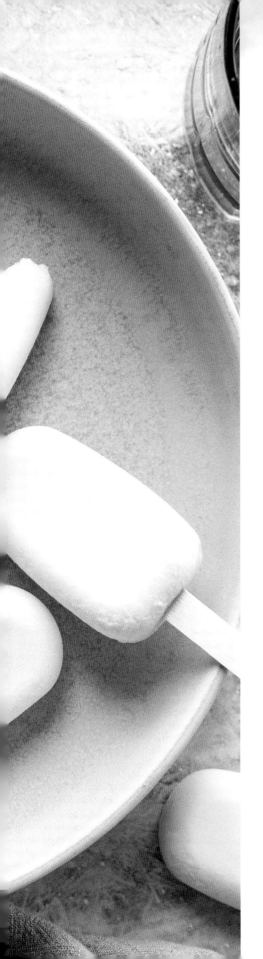

chapter 4

Desserts & Sweet Treats

Strawberry Pavlova / 232

Fudge Pops / 234

Electrolyte Ice Pops / 235

Orange Creamsicle Ice Pops / 236

Electrolyte Gummies / 238

Snow Cones / 240

Fruity Ice Pops / 241

Strawberry Protein Pops / 242

Strawberries and Cream Ice Pops / 243

Chocolate Meringue Cookies / 244

Strawberry Angel Food Cake / 246

Vanilla Angel Food Cupcakes / 248

Strawberry Shortcake / 250

Bread Pudding / 252

Tiramisu / 254

Boccone Dolce Cake / 256

Strawberry Pavlova

  yield: 4 servings • prep time: 10 minutes • cook time: 1 hour 20 minutes

Pavlova is a delicate meringue-based dessert that isn't overly sweet. Please note that meringue and humidity do not mix, so make this recipe on a day that isn't too humid. Otherwise, the exterior of your meringue shell will not be as crisp as it should be.

3 large egg whites

¼ teaspoon cream of tartar

¾ cup confectioners'-style erythritol

1 teaspoon strawberry extract

1. Preheat the oven to 275°F. Lightly grease a 7-inch pie plate with coconut oil spray.

2. In a medium-sized mixing bowl, beat the egg whites and cream of tartar with an electric hand mixer on high speed until soft peaks form. Add the sweetener in small increments and beat on low, mixing well after each addition. Add the strawberry extract. Increase the speed to high and continue to beat until stiff peaks form.

3. Spread the mixture on the bottom, up the sides, and onto the rim of the pie plate to form a shell. Bake for 1 hour, then turn off the oven and let the meringue stand in the oven for 20 minutes. Transfer to a cooling rack to cool completely.

4. Cut into wedges and serve. Store any leftovers in an airtight container in the refrigerator for up to 3 days.

P/E ratio **4.5** • calories **27** • fat **0.1g** • protein **5g** • carbs **1g** • fiber **0g**

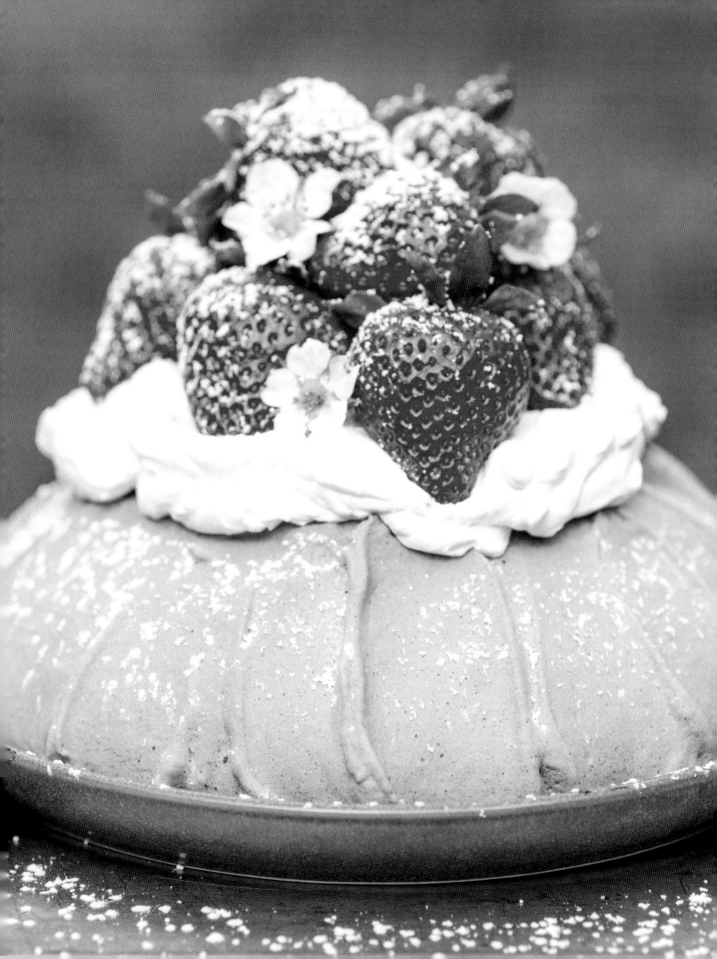

Fudge Pops

 yield: 8 fudge pops (1 per serving) • prep time: 5 minutes, plus overnight to freeze

10 large hard-boiled egg whites, or 1¼ cups 100% liquid egg whites, lightly scrambled

1 cup unsweetened almond milk or cashew milk

¼ cup confectioners'-style erythritol, or more to taste

2½ tablespoons unsweetened cocoa powder

2 teaspoons vanilla extract

½ teaspoon ground cinnamon

⅛ teaspoon fine sea salt

1. Put all of the ingredients in a blender and blend until very smooth. Taste and add more sweetener if needed.

2. Pour the mixture into 8 ice pop molds and insert the sticks. Freeze overnight, until solid. Store in the freezer for up to 1 month.

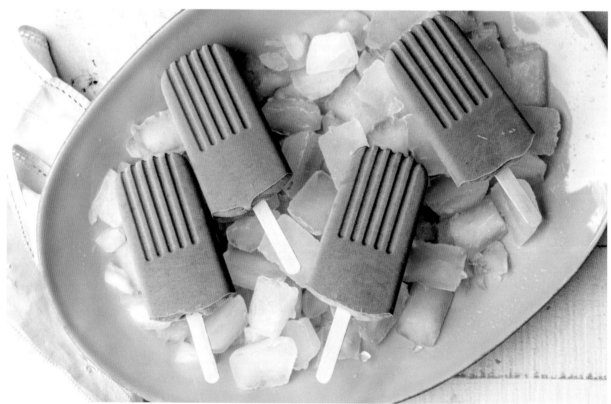

P/E ratio **3.1** • calories **32** • fat **1g** • protein **5g** • carbs **1g** • fiber **0.4g**

Electrolyte Ice Pops

   yield: 8 ice pops (1 per serving) • prep time: 5 minutes, plus overnight to freeze

2 tablespoons fruit-flavored zero-calorie electrolyte drink mix (or 2 packets LMNT electrolyte drink mix)

2 cups water

1. Combine the drink mix and water; stir until fully dissolved.

2. Pour into 8 ice pop molds, leaving room for expansion, and insert the sticks. Freeze overnight, until solid. Store in the freezer for up to 1 month.

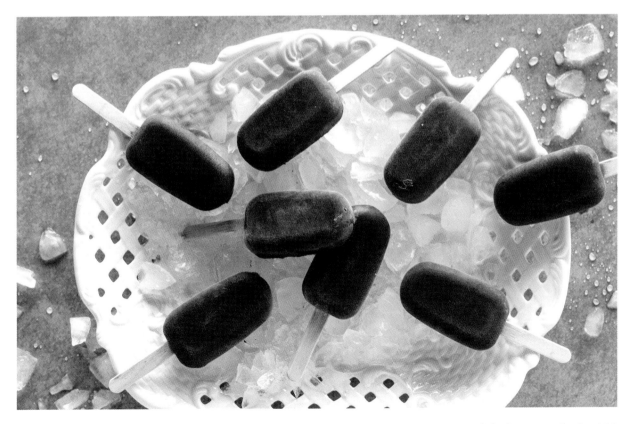

P/E ratio 0 • calories 5 • fat 0g • protein 0g • carbs 1g • fiber 0g

Orange Creamsicle
Ice Pops

 yield: 8 ice pops (1 per serving) • prep time: 5 minutes, plus overnight to freeze

10 large hard-boiled egg whites, or 1¼ cups 100% liquid egg whites, lightly scrambled

1 cup unsweetened almond milk or cashew milk

¼ cup confectioners'-style erythritol, plus more to taste

2 teaspoons orange extract

⅛ teaspoon orange-flavored liquid stevia

⅛ teaspoon fine sea salt

1. Put all of the ingredients in a blender and blend until very smooth. Taste and add more sweetener if needed.

2. Pour the mixture into 8 ice pop molds and insert the sticks. Freeze overnight, until solid. Store in the freezer for up to 1 month.

P/E ratio **7.1** • calories **25** • fat **0.4g** • protein **5g** • carbs **0.4g** • fiber **0.1g**

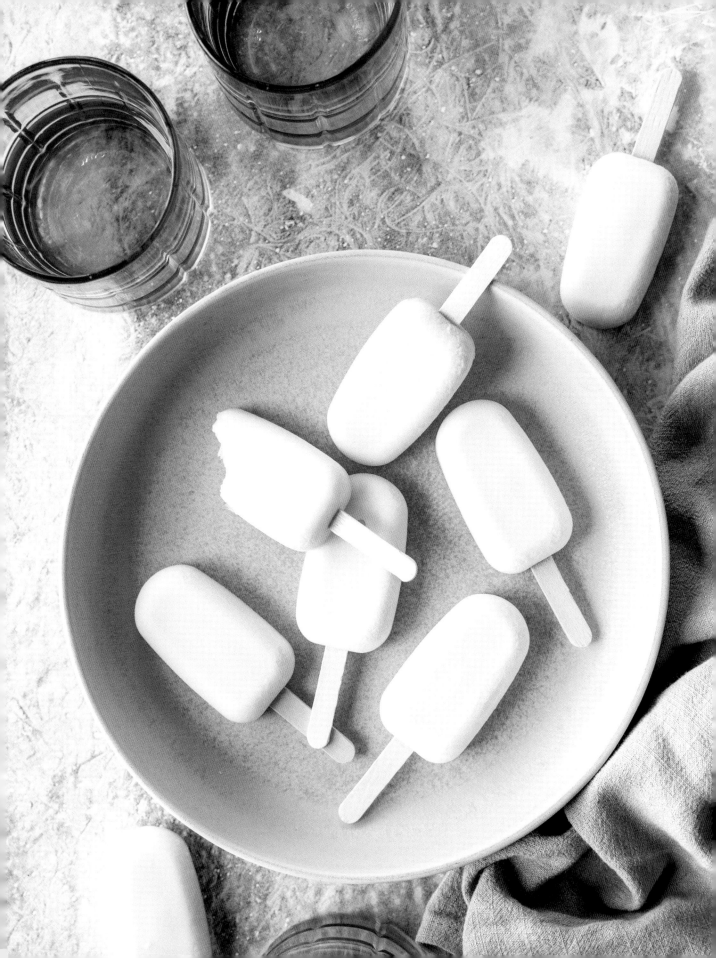

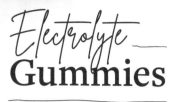

Electrolyte Gummies

    yield: 1 serving • prep time: 4 minutes, plus 2 hours to set • cook time: 2 minutes

Electrolytes are very helpful when you begin PSMF because they will help you combat low energy, low moods, constipation, and headaches. These gummies are a delicious salty-sweet chewy treat, and you can make them any flavor you want based on your choice of electrolyte drink mix.

½ cup water

1½ tablespoons grass-fed powdered gelatin

1 tablespoon zero-calorie electrolyte drink mix (or 1 packet LMNT electrolyte drink mix)

Special Equipment:

Silicone gummy tray

1. Put the water in a small saucepan. Whisk in the gelatin until softened. Whisk in the drink mix. Bring the mixture to a gentle boil over medium-high heat. Remove the pan from the heat.

2. Use a turkey baster to fill a silicone gummy tray with the mixture. Refrigerate until set, about 2 hours. (The longer the gummies sit in the refrigerator, the chewier they will be.) Store in the refrigerator for up to 6 days.

P/E ratio **4.0** • calories **48** • fat **0g** • protein **8g** • carbs **2g** • fiber **0g**

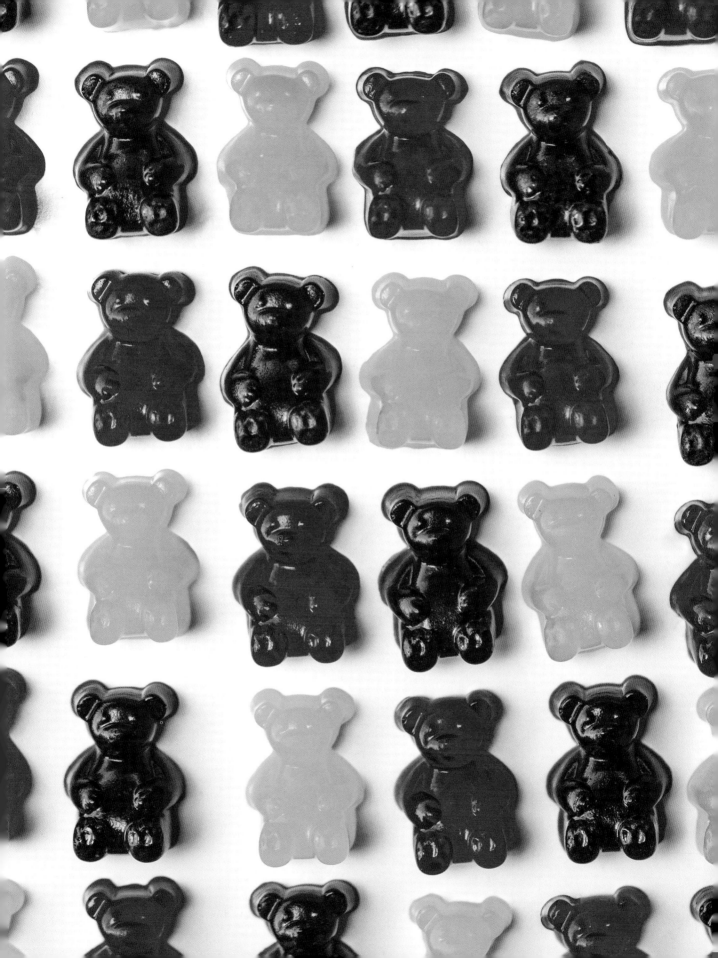

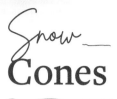

Snow Cones

    yield: 2 servings • prep time: 2 minutes

Hawaiians love their shaved ice; you can find shaved-ice vendors all over the islands. Here's everything we love about shaved ice without the food dye or the sugar. With a home shaved-ice machine, we make these snow cones at home every night, and so can you!

2 cups shaved ice

2 tablespoons any flavor zero-calorie electrolyte drink mix

¼ cup water

1. Divide the shaved ice between two cups.

2. Combine the drink mix and water; stir until fully dissolved. Drizzle over the ice and enjoy!

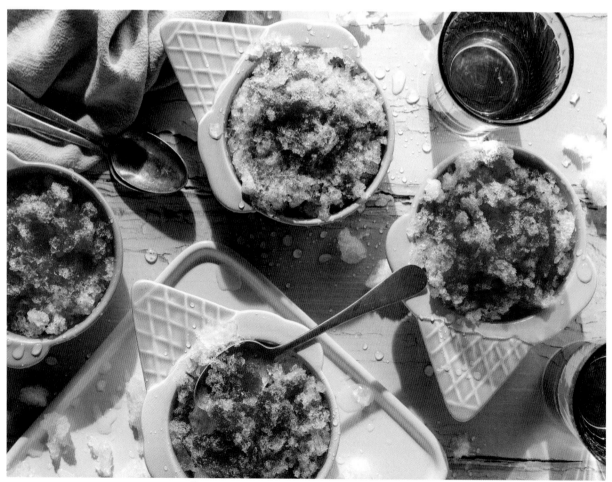

P/E ratio **0** • calories **0** • fat **0g** • protein **0g** • carbs **0g** • fiber **0g**

Fruity
Ice Pops

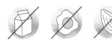 yield: 4 ice pops (1 per serving) • prep time: 5 minutes, plus 4 hours to freeze

My favorite fizzy water to use in this recipe is coconut-flavored LaCroix.

1 cup zero-calorie carbonated water or water

1½ teaspoons zero-calorie electrolyte drink mix (any flavor)

¼ teaspoon strawberry-flavored stevia or other fruit-flavored stevia, such as coconut

1. Put all of the ingredients in a blender and blend until very smooth.

2. Pour the mixture into 4 ice pop molds and insert the sticks. Freeze until solid, about 4 hours. Store in the freezer for up to 1 month.

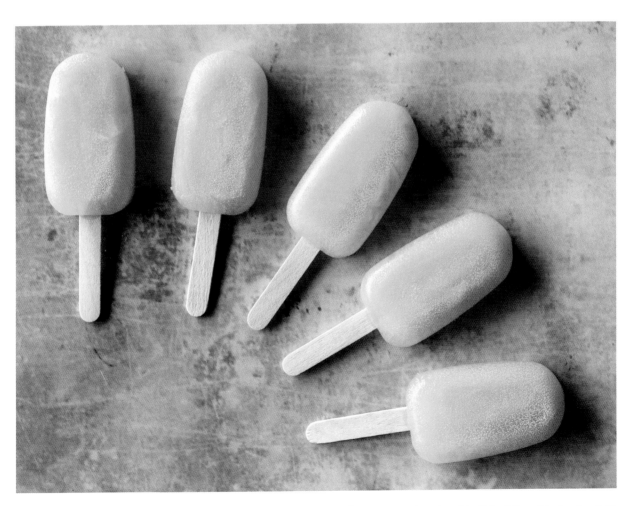

P/E ratio **0** • calories **0** • fat **0g** • protein **0g** • carbs **0g** • fiber **0g**   The Protein-Sparing Modified Fast Method   241

Strawberry Protein Pops

  yield: 4 ice pops (1 per serving) • prep time: 5 minutes, plus overnight to freeze

1 cup unsweetened almond milk or cashew milk

¼ cup vanilla-flavored beef protein powder

1 teaspoon strawberry extract

⅛ teaspoon strawberry-flavored liquid stevia, or more to taste

1. Put all of the ingredients in a blender and blend until very smooth. Taste and add more sweetener if needed.

2. Pour the mixture into 4 ice pop molds and insert the sticks. Freeze overnight, until solid. Store in the freezer for up to 1 month.

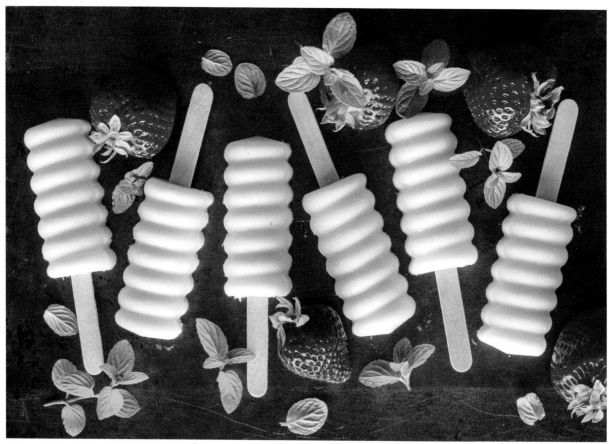

P/E ratio **4.2** • calories **29** • fat **1g** • protein **5g** • carbs **0.3g** • fiber **0.1g**

Strawberries and Cream
Ice Pops

 yield: 8 ice pops (1 per serving) • prep time: 5 minutes, plus overnight to freeze

10 large hard-boiled egg whites, or 1¼ cups 100% liquid egg whites, lightly scrambled

1 cup unsweetened almond milk or cashew milk

¼ cup confectioners'-style erythritol, or more to taste

2 teaspoons strawberry extract

⅛ teaspoon strawberry-flavored liquid stevia

⅛ teaspoon fine sea salt

1. Put all of the ingredients in a blender and blend until very smooth. Taste and add more sweetener if needed.

2. Pour the mixture into 8 ice pop molds and insert the sticks. Freeze overnight, until solid. Store in the freezer for up to 1 month.

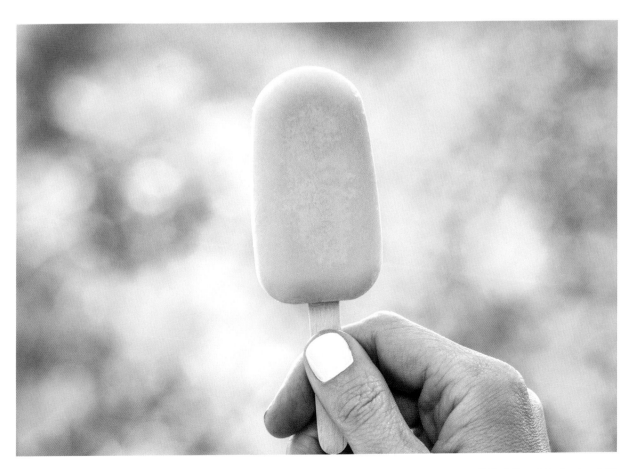

Chocolate
Meringue Cookies

  yield: 16 cookies (2 per serving) • prep time: 10 minutes • cook time: 1 hour 20 minutes

3 large egg whites

¼ teaspoon cream of tartar

¼ cup confectioners'-style erythritol

2 tablespoons unsweetened cocoa powder

1 teaspoon vanilla extract

1. Preheat the oven to 225°F. Line a baking sheet with parchment paper.

2. In a medium-sized mixing bowl, beat the egg whites and cream of tartar with an electric hand mixer on high speed until soft peaks form. Add the sweetener and cocoa powder in small increments and mix well on low speed after each addition. Add the vanilla extract and continue to beat on high until stiff peaks form.

3. Spoon the mixture into a piping bag and pipe 1-inch rounds onto the parchment, leaving about ¼ inch of space between them. Bake for 1 hour, then turn off the oven and let the cookies stand in the oven for another 20 minutes.

4. Transfer to a cooling rack to cool completely before enjoying. Store extras in an airtight container for up to 6 days.

P/E ratio **2.0** • calories **12** • fat **0.3g** • protein **2g** • carbs **1g** • fiber **0.3g**

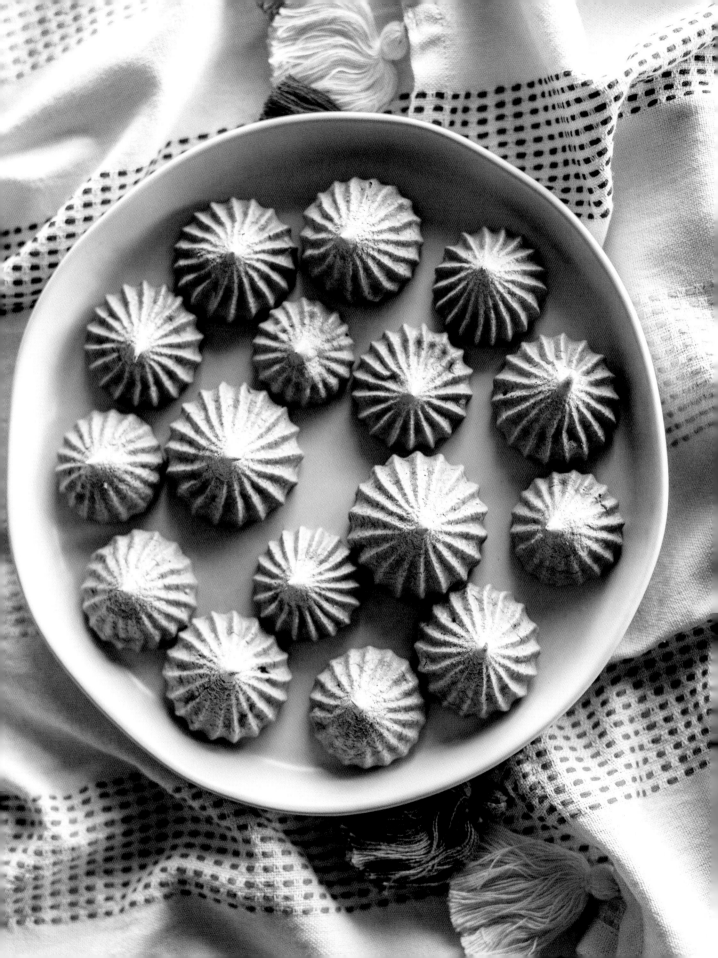

Strawberry Angel Food Cake

  yield: one 10-inch cake (12 servings) • prep time: 10 minutes • cook time: 45 minutes

Not only does this angel food cake taste great on its own, but it also makes the most delicious French toast (see page 76).

Coconut oil spray, for greasing

1 cup unflavored egg white protein powder

1 cup confectioners'-style erythritol

12 large egg whites

Pinch of fine sea salt

2 teaspoons cream of tartar

2 teaspoons strawberry extract

Special Equipment:

10-inch tube pan

Variation: ————

Classic Angel Food Cake. *Simply replace the strawberry extract with an equal amount of vanilla extract.*

1. Preheat the oven to 350°F. Lightly grease a 10-inch tube pan with coconut oil spray.

2. Sift the protein powder and sweetener together; set aside.

3. In a large clean bowl, beat the egg whites and salt with an electric hand mixer on high speed until foamy. Add the cream of tartar and continue to beat until stiff peaks form.

4. Gently fold in the protein powder mixture and strawberry extract, being careful not to deflate the egg whites. Pour the batter into the prepared pan. Bake until a toothpick inserted into the center comes out clean, about 45 minutes.

5. Let the cake cool completely in the pan before unmolding. Cut into 12 slices and serve. Store leftover cake in an airtight container in the refrigerator for up to 6 days or in the freezer for up to 1 month.

P/E ratio **9.1** • calories **47** • fat **0.1g** • protein **10g** • carbs **1g** • fiber **0g**

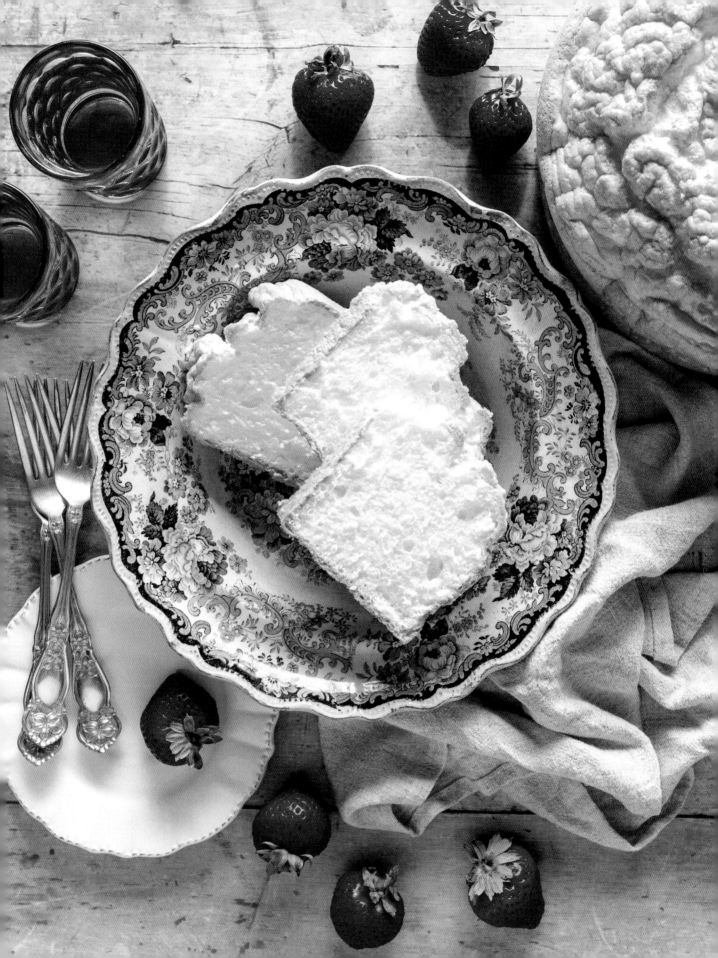

Vanilla Angel Food Cupcakes

  yield: 12 cupcakes (1 per serving) • prep time: 20 minutes, plus time to cool • cook time: 20 minutes

Coconut oil spray, for greasing

1 cup unflavored egg white protein powder

1 cup confectioners'-style erythritol

12 large egg whites

Pinch of fine sea salt

2 teaspoons cream of tartar

2 teaspoons vanilla extract

Frosting:

2 large egg whites

1½ cups confectioners'-style erythritol

¼ teaspoon cream of tartar

⅓ cup cold water

1½ teaspoons vanilla extract

1. Preheat the oven to 350°F. Lightly grease a standard-size 12-well muffin pan with coconut oil spray.

2. Sift the protein powder and sweetener together; set aside.

3. In a large bowl, beat the egg whites and salt with an electric hand mixer on high speed until foamy. Add the cream of tartar and continue to beat until very stiff peaks form. Gently fold in the protein powder mixture and vanilla extract, being careful not to deflate the egg whites.

4. Divide the batter evenly among the wells of the prepared muffin pan. Bake until a toothpick inserted in the center of a cupcake comes out clean, about 20 minutes. Let cool completely in the pan.

5. When the cupcakes are almost completely cool, make the frosting: Fill a medium-sized saucepan one-third of the way with water. Put all of the ingredients in a large metal bowl that fits on top of the saucepan without its bottom touching the water. Set the pan over medium-high heat and bring to a boil; lower the heat to get the water gently simmering.

6. Beat the egg white mixture with an electric hand mixer on high speed until thickened, about 7 minutes. Remove the bowl from the saucepan and continue to beat the mixture off the heat until stiff peaks form. Use immediately to frost the cooled cupcakes.

P/E ratio **9.1** • calories **54** • fat **0.1g** • protein **10g** • carbs **1g** • fiber **0g**

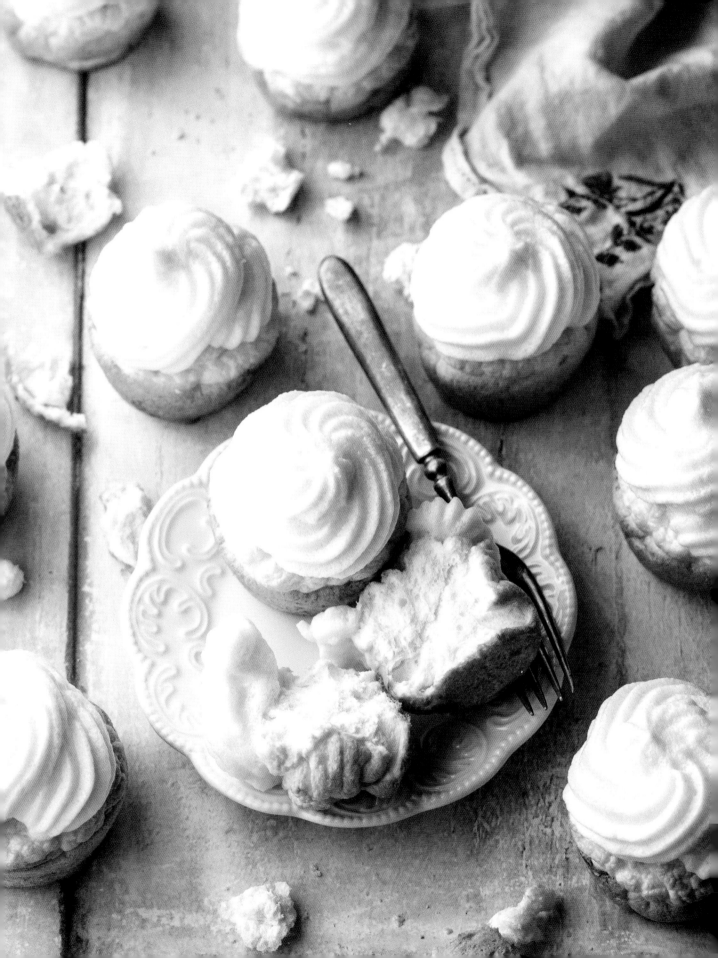

Strawberry Shortcake

 yield: 12 servings • prep time: 10 minutes (not including time to make cake)

This is a dairy-free, high-protein, low-fat twist on my son Micah's favorite dessert. This protein-sparing version does not disappoint. It is creamy and delicious!

1 Strawberry Angel Food Cake (page 246)

10 large hard-boiled egg whites, or 1¼ cups 100% liquid egg whites, lightly scrambled

1 cup unsweetened almond milk or cashew milk

¼ cup confectioners'-style erythritol

2 teaspoons vanilla or strawberry extract

⅛ teaspoon fine sea salt

6 strawberries, thinly sliced, for garnish (optional)

1. Cut the cake into 12 slices.

2. Put the egg whites, milk, sweetener, extract, and salt in a blender and blend until very smooth.

3. Top each slice of cake with a dollop of the egg white mixture. Garnish with a few strawberry slices, if desired, and serve immediately.

P/E ratio **1.6** • calories **27** • fat **0.2g** • protein **3g** • carbs **2g** • fiber **0.3g**

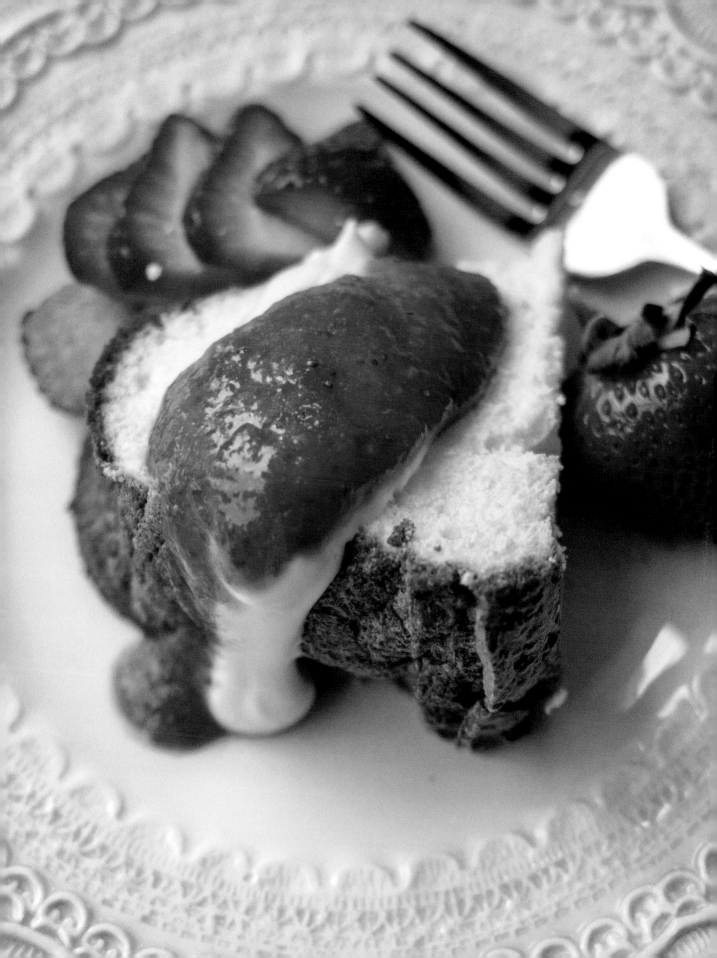

Bread Pudding

yield: 12 servings • prep time: 10 minutes (not including time to make bread) • cook time: 45 minutes (25 minutes if using a muffin pan)

Coconut oil spray, for greasing

1 loaf Protein-Sparing Bread (page 270), cut into 1-inch cubes

8 large egg whites

1 cup unsweetened almond milk or cashew milk

1 teaspoon vanilla extract

⅔ cup confectioners'-style erythritol

1 teaspoon ground cinnamon

½ teaspoon fine sea salt

Glaze:

1 cup confectioners'-style erythritol

½ teaspoon vanilla or strawberry extract

3 to 4 tablespoons unsweetened almond milk or cashew milk

1. Preheat the oven to 350°F. Grease a 7 by 11-inch baking dish or a standard-size 12-well muffin pan with duck fat spray or coconut oil spray.

2. Put the bread cubes in a large bowl. In a medium-sized bowl, combine the egg whites, milk, vanilla extract, sweetener, cinnamon, and salt; blend well. Pour the egg mixture over the bread and mix well; transfer to the prepared baking dish or muffin pan (if using a muffin pan, fill each well about two-thirds full).

3. Bake until set, 45 minutes to 1 hour if using a baking dish or 25 to 30 minutes if using a muffin pan. Allow to cool completely in the dish or pan.

4. Meanwhile, make the glaze: Put the sweetener and extract in a small bowl. Stir in the milk, 1 tablespoon at a time, until you have a spreadable glaze. Add more milk if you prefer a thinner glaze.

5. If you used a baking dish, cut the bread pudding into 12 equal pieces. Drizzle 1 to 2 tablespoons of the glaze over each piece and serve. Store leftovers in an airtight container in the refrigerator for up to 3 days.

P/E ratio 2.1 • calories 58 • fat 3g • protein 7g • carbs 0.4g • fiber 0.1g

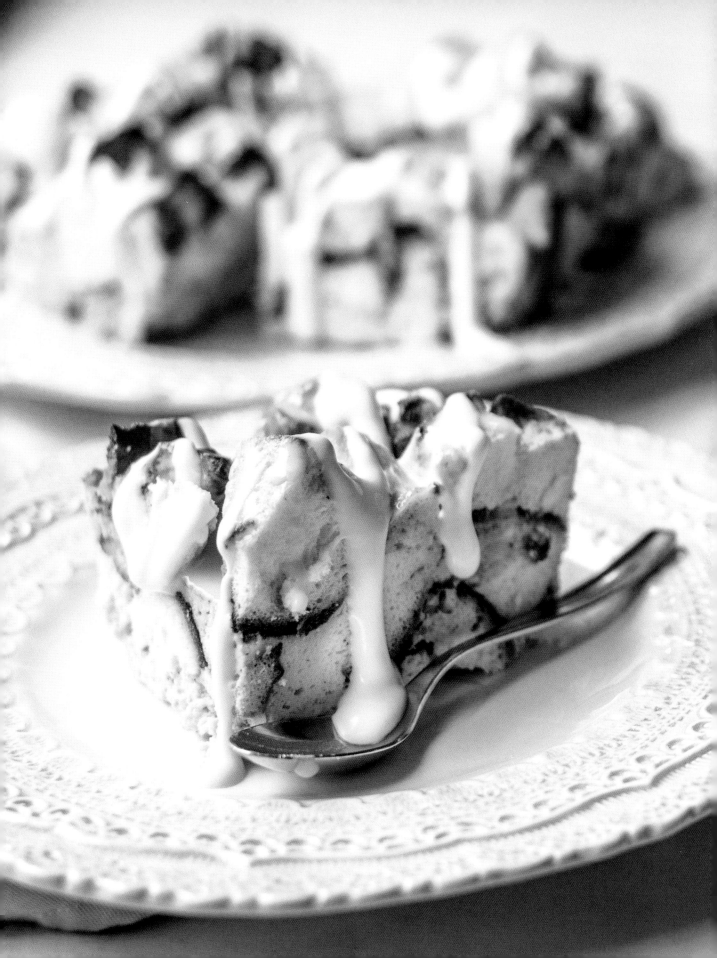

Tiramisu

 yield: 12 servings • prep time: 15 minutes, plus 1 hour to refrigerate (not including time to make bread)

This is a dairy-free, high-protein, low-fat twist on my favorite dessert. I usually do not drink caffeine, but the small amount in a serving of this delicious dessert is totally worth it. You can also use Classic Angel Food Cake (page 246) in place of the protein-sparing bread to make the ladyfingers, but the dessert will be much sweeter.

½ loaf Protein-Sparing Bread (page 270)

¾ cup brewed decaf espresso or strong brewed decaf coffee

½ cup confectioners'-style erythritol, divided

3 teaspoons rum extract, divided

½ teaspoon vanilla extract

10 large hard-boiled egg whites, or 1¼ cups 100% liquid egg whites, lightly scrambled

1 cup unsweetened almond milk or cashew milk

⅛ teaspoon fine sea salt

2 tablespoons unsweetened cocoa powder, divided

1. Cut the crust off the bread and slice the bread into 18 strips, about 1 inch wide and 4 inches long. Set aside.

2. In a small bowl, mix the espresso, ¼ cup of the sweetener, 1 teaspoon of the rum extract, and the vanilla extract until well combined. Set aside.

3. Make the filling: Put the egg whites, milk, the remaining ¼ cup of sweetener, the remaining 2 teaspoons of rum extract, and the salt in a blender; blend until very smooth. Taste and adjust the sweetness to your liking.

4. Arrange 6 bread strips, flat side down (they absorb more coffee dip that way), in a 2-quart baking dish or an 8-inch square baking pan. Drizzle 1 teaspoon of the coffee mixture over each strip. Layer one-third of the filling over the bread. Dust with about one-quarter of the cocoa powder. Repeat this process twice more, ending with the remaining cocoa powder. Cover and refrigerate for at least 1 hour or up to 3 days to set.

5. Cut into 12 pieces and serve.

P/E ratio **5.4** • calories **39** • fat **0.4g** • protein **7g** • carbs **1g** • fiber **0.1g**

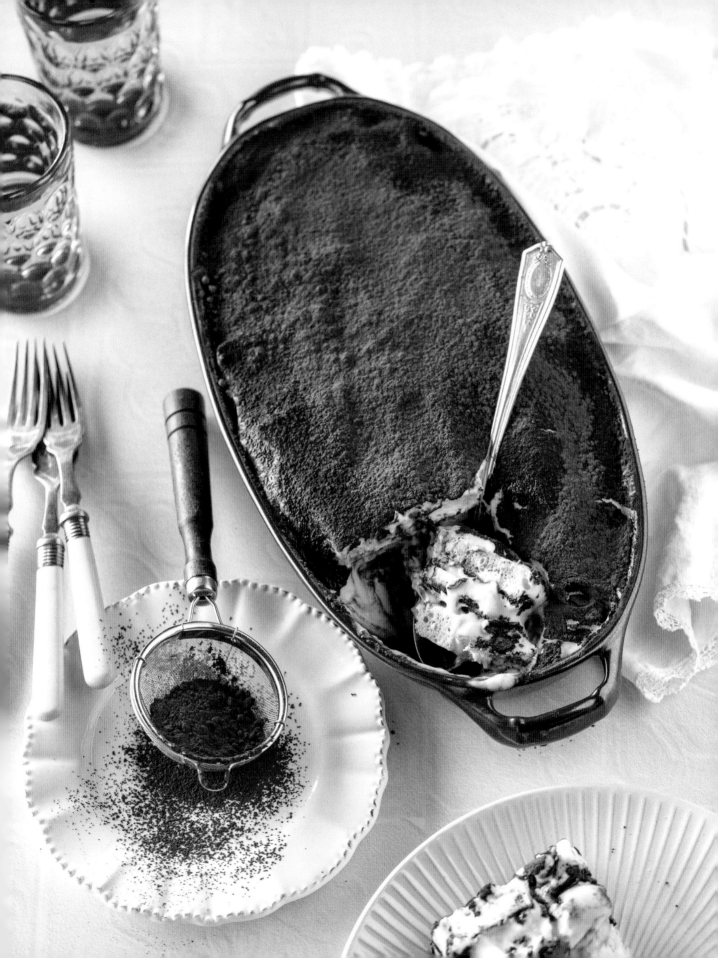

Boccone
Dolce Cake

 yield: 10 servings • prep time: 15 minutes • cook time: 3 hours 20 minutes

Boccone dolce ("sweet mouthful") is a stunning Italian meringue-based layered dessert. Just make sure to take a photo before you slice it since it crumbles!

Cake:

10 large egg whites, room temperature

1¼ cups confectioners'-style erythritol

¼ teaspoon cream of tartar

¼ teaspoon fine sea salt

Filling:

10 large hard-boiled egg whites, or 1¼ cups 100% liquid egg whites, lightly scrambled

1 cup unsweetened almond milk

½ cup confectioners'-style erythritol, or more to taste

2½ tablespoons unsweetened cocoa powder

2 teaspoons vanilla extract

⅛ teaspoon fine sea salt

Chocolate Drizzle:

⅓ cup unsweetened almond milk

½ cup confectioners'-style erythritol

3 ounces unsweetened baking chocolate, finely chopped

1 teaspoon vanilla extract

⅛ teaspoon fine sea salt

1. Preheat the oven to 200°F. Cut out three 9-inch rounds of parchment paper and place them on two large baking sheets.

2. Make the cake: In a large bowl, beat the egg whites, sweetener, cream of tartar, and salt with an electric hand mixer on high speed until stiff peaks form, 5 to 7 minutes. Evenly divide the meringue mixture between the three parchment rounds and spread each portion into a 1-inch-high disk, flattening the top and making sure it is smooth and even. Bake for 3 hours, then turn off the oven, letting the residual heat continue to bake them for another 20 minutes. Transfer the meringue disks to a wire rack to cool completely.

3. Meanwhile, make the filling: Put all of the filling ingredients in a blender and puree until very smooth. Taste and add more sweetener if needed. Transfer to a bowl, cover, and keep refrigerated while the meringue disks are cooling.

4. Just before assembly, make the chocolate drizzle: Put the almond milk and sweetener in a small saucepan and bring to a gentle boil over medium heat. Remove the pan from the heat and stir in the chocolate, vanilla extract, and salt. Let sit for 3 minutes, then stir again until completely smooth.

5. Assemble the cake: Once the meringue disks have cooled completely, peel off the parchment and place one disk on a cake plate. Using a spatula, spread one-third of the filling on the meringue. Drizzle one-third of the chocolate over the filling. Repeat with the remaining meringue disks, filling, and chocolate drizzle.

6. Cut into slices with a very sharp knife and serve. Store leftovers in an airtight container in the refrigerator for up to 3 days.

P/E ratio **1.1** • calories **107** • fat **6g** • protein **9g** • carbs **4g** • fiber **2g**

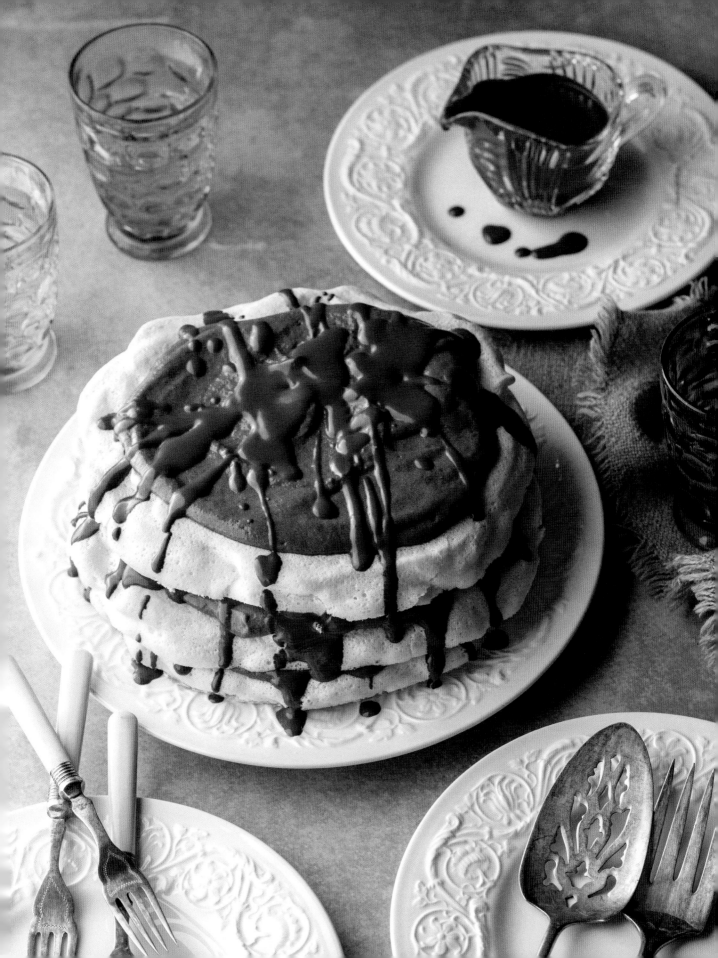

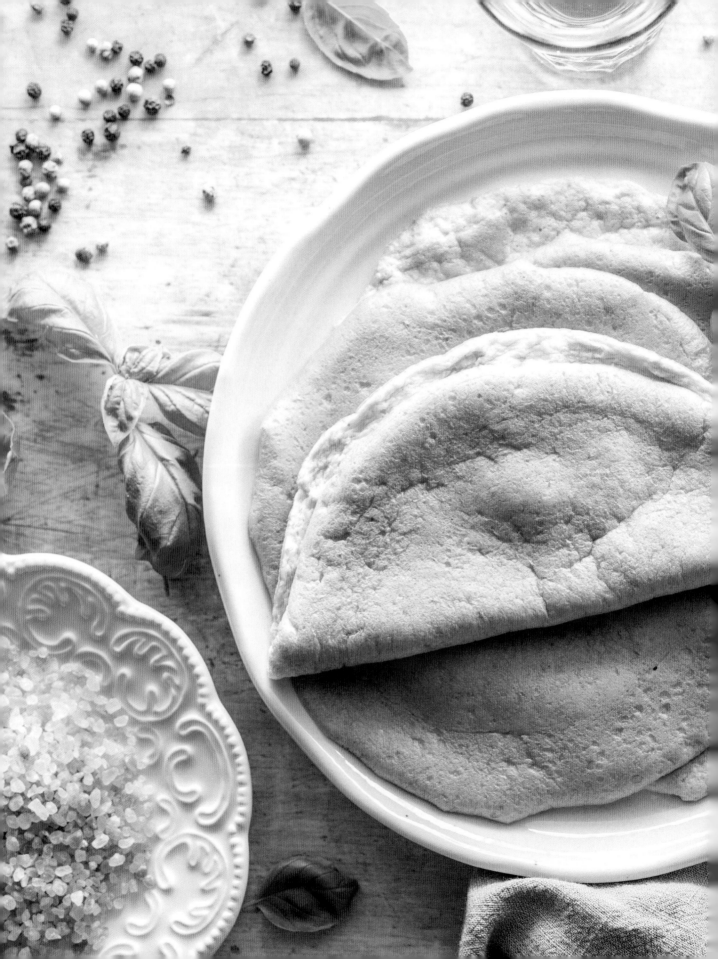

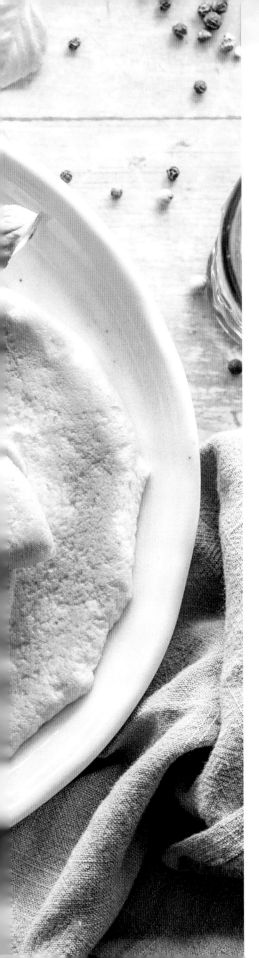

chapter 5

Sauces & Basics

Chimichurri Sauce / 260

Orange Marmalade / 262

Spicy BBQ Vinegar Sauce / 264

Dijon Vinaigrette / 266

Carolina BBQ Sauce / 267

Cilantro Lime Sauce / 268

Mayo / 269

Protein-Sparing Bread / 270

Protein-Sparing Waffle Buns / 272

Basil Wraps / 274

Chimichurri
Sauce

   yield: 2 cups (2 tablespoons per serving) • prep time: 5 minutes, plus 1 hour to rest

This protein-sparing adaptation of the popular herbaceous, garlicky sauce from Argentina is great not only with steak but also with chicken, fish, or seafood.

1 cup packed fresh flat-leaf parsley leaves

¾ cup apple cider vinegar

¼ cup packed fresh cilantro leaves

3 cloves garlic, peeled

¾ teaspoon red pepper flakes

½ teaspoon ground cumin

½ teaspoon fine sea salt

1. Put all of the ingredients in a food processor and puree until smooth. Transfer to a serving bowl.

2. Cover and let stand at room temperature for about 1 hour to allow the flavors to meld. Store in an airtight container in the refrigerator for up to 2 weeks.

P/E ratio **0.7** • calories **2** • fat **0g** • protein **0.2g** • carbs **0.5g** • fiber **0.2g**

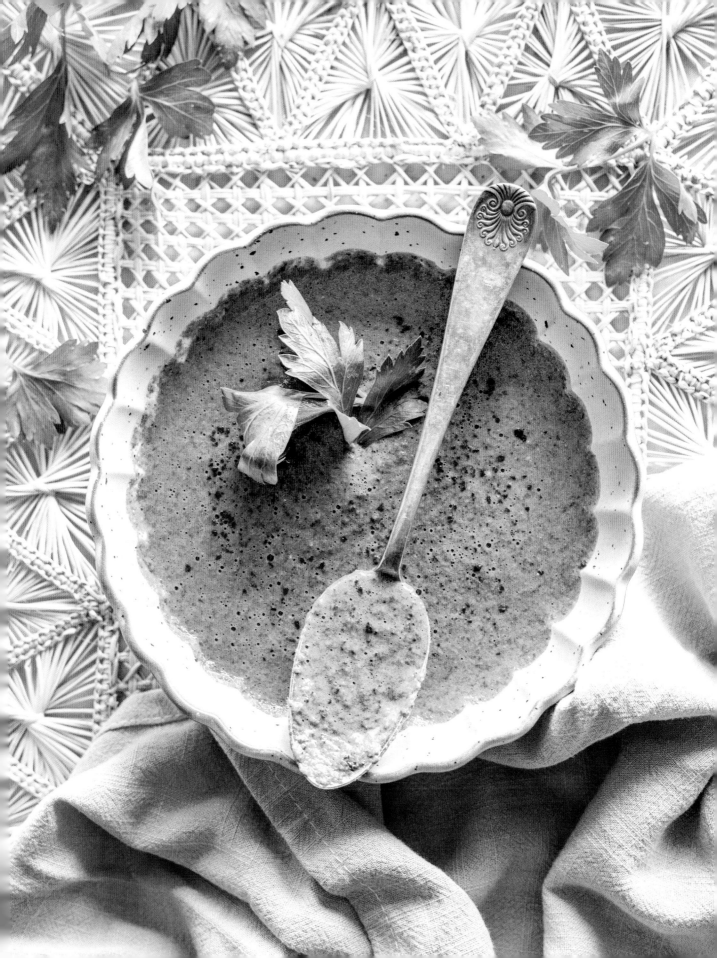

Orange Marmalade

   yield: 1½ cups (2 tablespoons per serving) • prep time: 2 minutes, plus 2 hours to cool and set • cook time: 3 minutes

I enjoy this marmalade on slices of Protein-Sparing Bread (page 270) and use it in my Orange Chicken recipe (page 142). You can also use this recipe to make other fruit-flavored jellies: simply replace the orange extract with the extract of your choice and choose any fruit-flavored drink mix that pairs well with it.

Feel free to use any zero-calorie fruit-flavored drink mix you like. I recommend Everly brand drink mix, especially the peach mango flavor, which gives the marmalade just the right flavor and color. If you use Everly, omit the citric acid powder.

1 cup cold water

2 teaspoons grass-fed powdered gelatin

2 tablespoons confectioners'-style erythritol, or more to taste

2 teaspoons orange extract

⅛ teaspoon citric acid powder

1 teaspoon zero-calorie orange drink mix

1. Put the water in a small saucepan. Sprinkle the gelatin into the water and allow it to soften for a few minutes.

2. Bring the water to a boil over high heat, then immediately remove the pan from the heat. Stir in the sweetener. Taste and add more sweetener if needed.

3. Add the orange extract, citric acid powder, and drink mix; stir to combine. Let sit on the counter to cool and set for at least 2 hours before using. Store in a jar in the refrigerator for up to 5 days.

P/E ratio **0** • calories **1** • fat **0g** • protein **0.3g** • carbs **0g** • fiber **0g**

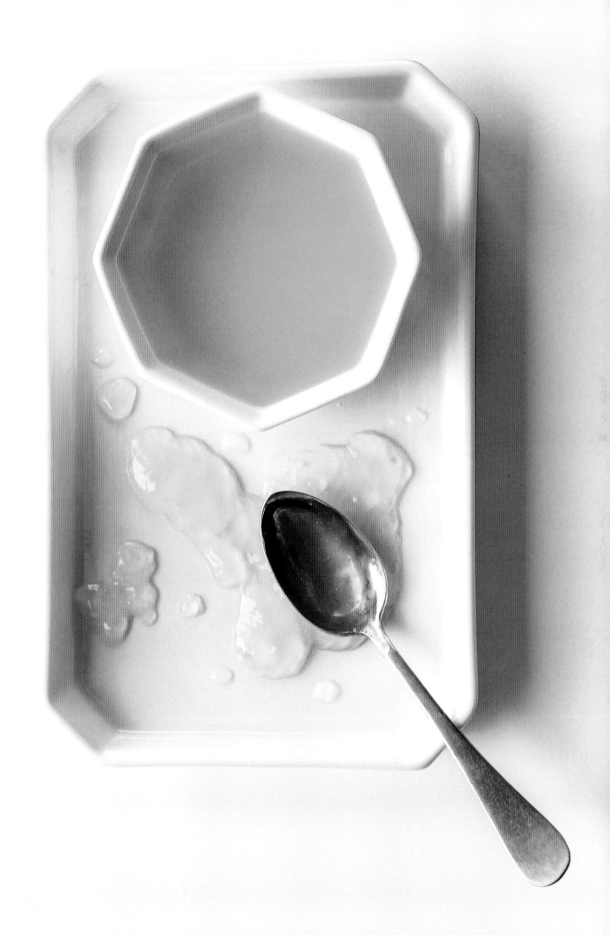

Spicy BBQ Vinegar Sauce

   yield: 2¼ cups (2 tablespoons per serving) • prep time: 2 minutes

This spicy sauce tastes great with chicken, pork chops, or a juicy steak.

2 cups apple cider vinegar

3 tablespoons tomato sauce

1 tablespoon hot sauce

2 tablespoons smoked paprika

2 tablespoons brown sugar–style erythritol, or more to taste

4 teaspoons smoked salt, or 4 teaspoons plain fine sea salt plus ⅛ teaspoon liquid smoke

1 teaspoon cayenne pepper, or more to taste

1 teaspoon freshly ground black pepper

Put all of the ingredients in a nonreactive mixing bowl and stir until the sweetener and salt have dissolved. Taste and add more sweetener and/or cayenne if needed. Store in a jar in the refrigerator for up to 2 weeks.

P/E ratio **0.1** • calories **3** • fat **0.1g** • protein **0.1g** • carbs **1g** • fiber **0.3g**

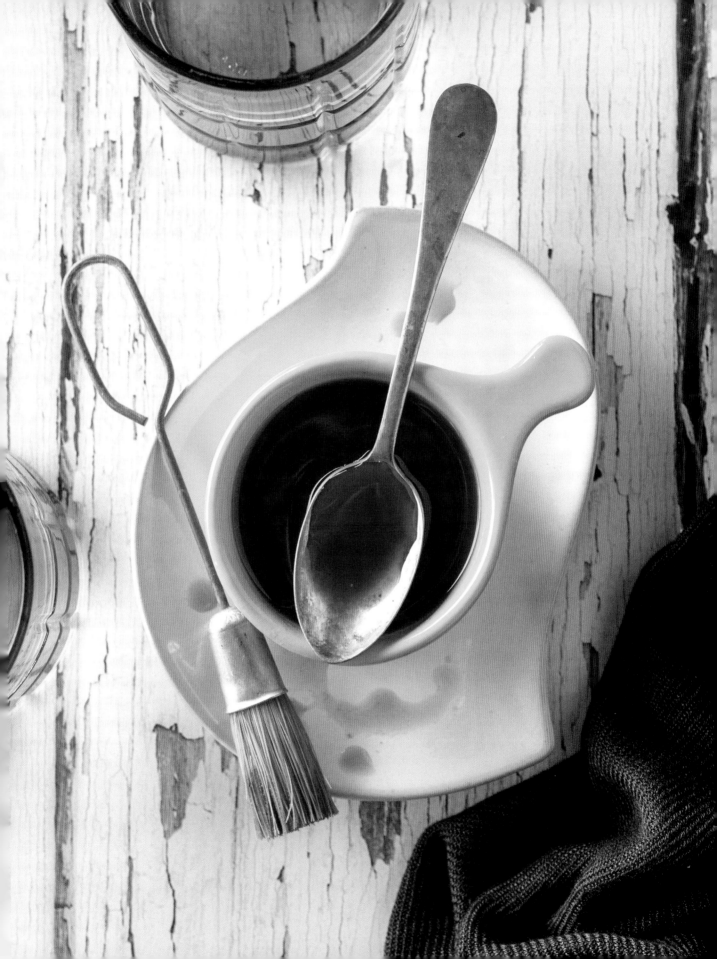

Dijon Vinaigrette

   yield: 1½ cups (1½ tablespoons per serving) • prep time: 5 minutes

½ cup fresh lemon juice

½ cup Dijon mustard

½ cup apple cider vinegar

4 cloves garlic, minced

Fine sea salt and freshly ground black pepper

In a medium-sized bowl, whisk together the lemon juice, mustard, vinegar, and garlic until well combined. Season with salt and pepper to taste. Store in a jar in the refrigerator for up to 2 weeks.

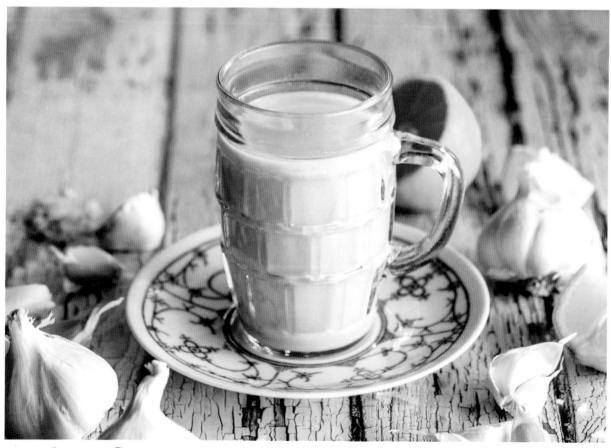

P/E ratio **0.1** • calories **10** • fat **0g** • protein **0.1g** • carbs **1g** • fiber **0.1g**

Carolina
BBQ Sauce

   yield: 2 cups (2 tablespoons per serving) • prep time: 5 minutes

1 cup prepared yellow mustard

¾ cup coconut vinegar or apple cider vinegar

2 tablespoons coconut oil (preferably butter-flavored), melted

1 teaspoon liquid smoke

⅛ teaspoon liquid stevia

1 tablespoon chili powder

1 teaspoon freshly ground black pepper

1 teaspoon freshly ground white pepper

¼ teaspoon cayenne pepper

Put all of the ingredients in a medium-sized bowl and stir until smooth. Store in a jar in the refrigerator for up to 2 weeks.

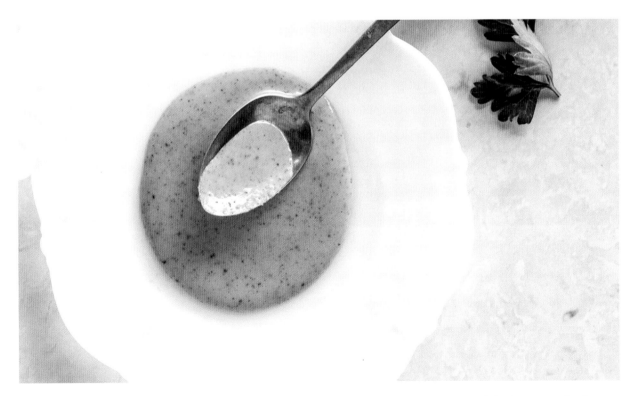

P/E ratio **0.1** • calories **36** • fat **3g** • protein **0.4g** • carbs **2g** • fiber **1g** The Protein-Sparing Modified Fast Method

Cilantro Lime Sauce

   yield: 1 cup (¼ cup per serving) • prep time: 5 minutes

¼ cup chicken broth

¼ cup fresh cilantro leaves

¼ cup lime juice

1 teaspoon minced garlic

1 teaspoon fine sea salt

½ teaspoon ground cumin

½ to 1 small jalapeño pepper, deseeded and sliced

Place all of the ingredients in a food processor and puree until smooth. Store in a jar in the refrigerator for up to 1 week.

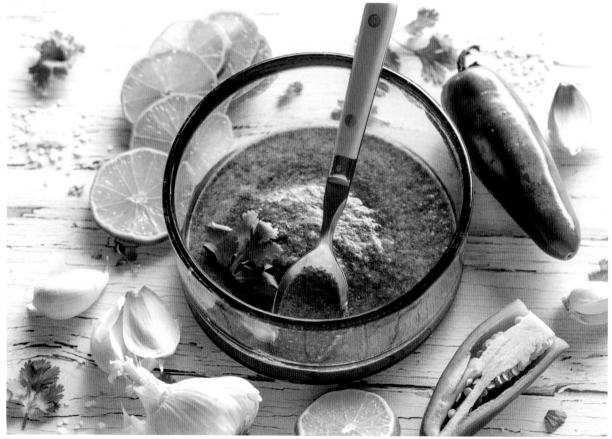

P/E ratio **0.5** • calories **9** • fat **0.1g** • protein **1g** • carbs **2g** • fiber **0.2g**

Mayo

  yield: 1½ cups (2 tablespoons per serving) • prep time: 5 minutes

6 large hard-boiled egg whites, or ¾ cup 100% liquid egg whites, lightly scrambled

¼ cup beef broth

1 teaspoon prepared yellow mustard

½ teaspoon apple cider vinegar or lemon juice

½ teaspoon fine sea salt

¼ teaspoon fish sauce (optional)

Put all of the ingredients in a wide-mouth jar and use an immersion blender to puree until completely smooth, scraping down the sides as needed with a small rubber spatula. Store in an airtight container in the refrigerator for up to 1 week.

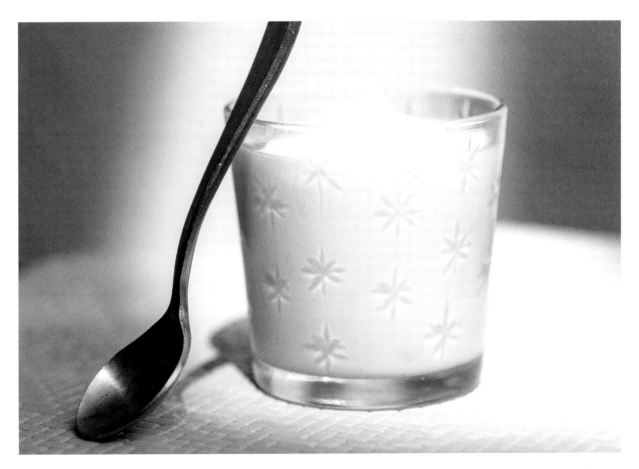

P/E ratio **1.4** • calories **37** • fat **2g** • protein **3g** • carbs **0.2g** • fiber **0g**   The Protein-Sparing Modified Fast Method

Protein-Sparing Bread

  yield: one 9 by 5-inch loaf (14 slices, 2 slices per serving) • prep time: 15 minutes, plus time to cool and 2 hours to rest • cook time: 40 minutes

This recipe produces a light, fluffy bread with a texture that's often compared to that of Wonder Bread. I often keep this bread in my refrigerator or freezer for easy additions to meals.

The keys are to use real egg whites, not liquid whites that come in a carton (which could cause the bread to fall), and to whip the heck out of them until they are very stiff—so stiff that the peaks stand straight up when you lift the beaters (you should be able to hold the bowl upside down and the egg whites stay put). If the peaks fold over themselves, keep beating, or you'll end up with something that's more like an eggy soufflé than bread.

Making this bread on a day that isn't too humid also helps, as meringues and humidity do not mix. Lastly, be sure to let the bread cool completely before slicing it or it will collapse.

Coconut oil spray, for greasing

12 large egg whites

1 teaspoon fine sea salt

½ teaspoon cream of tartar

1 cup unflavored egg white protein powder

Variation:

Cinnamon Protein-Sparing Bread. *Use a spatula to swirl 1½ tablespoons of ground cinnamon into the egg white mixture in step 3. This variation is great for making French toast (see page 74).*

1. Preheat the oven to 350°F. Lightly grease a 9 by 5-inch loaf pan with coconut oil spray.

2. Put the egg whites, salt, and cream of tartar in a large, grease-free bowl. Beat with an electric handheld mixer on high speed until very stiff peaks form, about 10 minutes. (You can also use a stand mixer fitted with the whisk attachment.)

3. Using a rubber spatula, slowly fold in the protein powder, being careful not to deflate the whites. (Do not overmix at this stage, or the bread will be stiff like Styrofoam!)

4. Transfer the batter to the prepared loaf pan and level out the top. Bake until golden brown, 40 to 45 minutes. Turn off the oven but leave the bread in the oven to cool completely.

5. Remove the cooled bread from the oven and leave it out on the kitchen counter for 2 hours before removing it from the pan and slicing. Store leftover bread in an airtight container in the refrigerator for up to 6 days or in the freezer for up to 1 month.

P/E ratio **14.0** • calories **79** • fat **0.1g** • protein **17g** • carbs **1g** • fiber **0g**

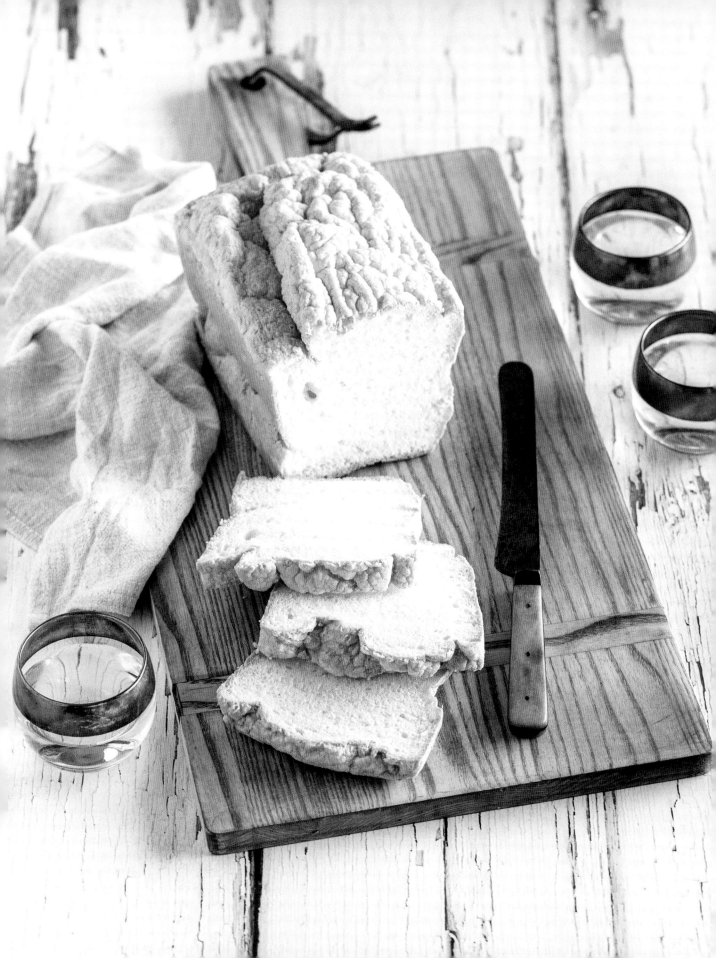

Protein-Sparing Waffle Buns

  yield: 2 buns (1 serving) • prep time: 4 minutes • cook time: 4 minutes

These mini waffles make perfect buns for a hamburger or sandwich. They're packed with protein and delicious!

1 large egg white

1 tablespoon unflavored egg white protein powder

⅛ teaspoon onion powder, garlic powder, everything bagel seasoning, or Italian seasoning (optional)

Coconut oil spray, for greasing

Special Equipment:

Mini waffle maker

1. Preheat a mini waffle maker.

2. Put the egg white in a medium-sized bowl and beat with an electric hand mixer on high speed until stiff peaks form. Add the protein powder and onion powder, if using; mix on low just until well combined, being careful not to deflate the whites.

3. Spray the waffle maker with coconut oil spray. Spoon half of the batter into the center and cook until firm and golden brown, 2 to 3 minutes. Repeat with the remaining batter.

4. Use right away, or store in an airtight container in the refrigerator for up to 4 days or in the freezer for up to 2 months.

P/E ratio **16.0** • calories **39** • fat **0.1g** • protein **8g** • carbs **0.4g** • fiber **0g**

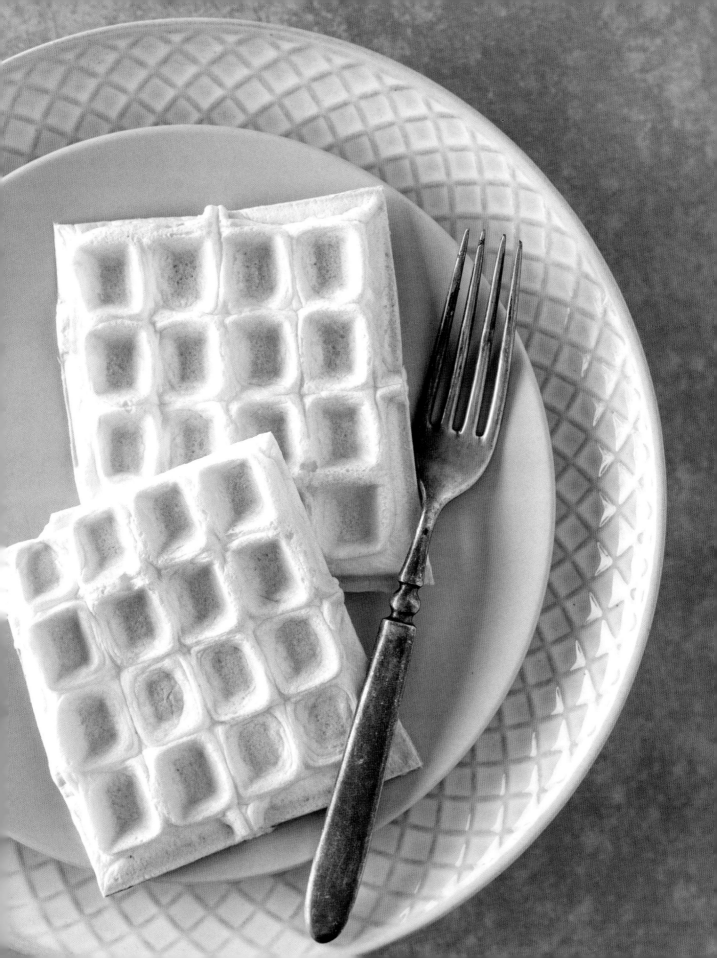

Basil Wraps

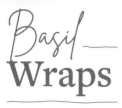 yield: 4 wraps (1 per serving) • prep time: 5 minutes • cook time: 12 minutes

These wraps are great for making sandwiches. You can also use this batter to make small waffles. Simply prepare the batter as instructed below and cook it in a mini waffle maker.

4 ounces extra-lean ground chicken

4 large egg whites

2 tablespoons chopped fresh basil leaves

½ teaspoon fine sea salt

Duck fat spray or coconut oil spray, for greasing

1. Place the ground chicken, egg whites, herbs, and salt in a blender; blend until very smooth.

2. Heat an 8-inch nonstick crepe pan or other skillet over medium-low heat. Lightly grease the pan with duck fat spray. When hot, pour one-quarter of the batter into the pan. Tilt the pan so the batter evenly covers the entire cooking surface. Cook, without flipping, until the batter sets and is cooked through, 3 to 4 minutes. Slide the wrap onto a plate to cool. Repeat with the remaining batter to make 4 wraps.

3. Store extras in an airtight container in the refrigerator for up to 3 days.

P/E ratio **9.2** • calories **57** • fat **1g** • protein **11g** • carbs **0.2g** • fiber **0g**

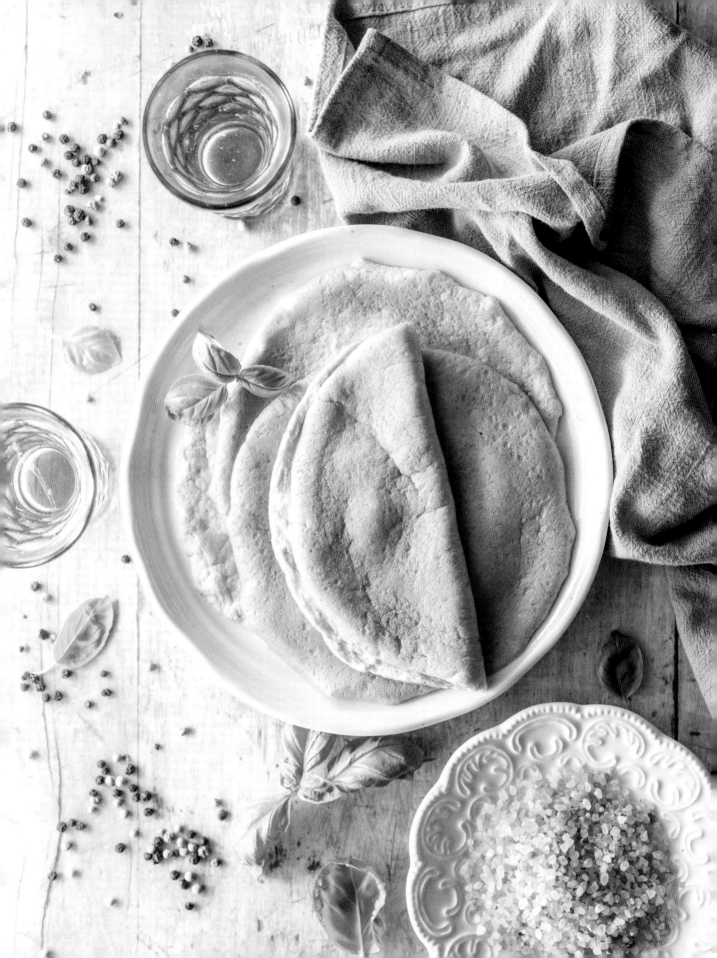

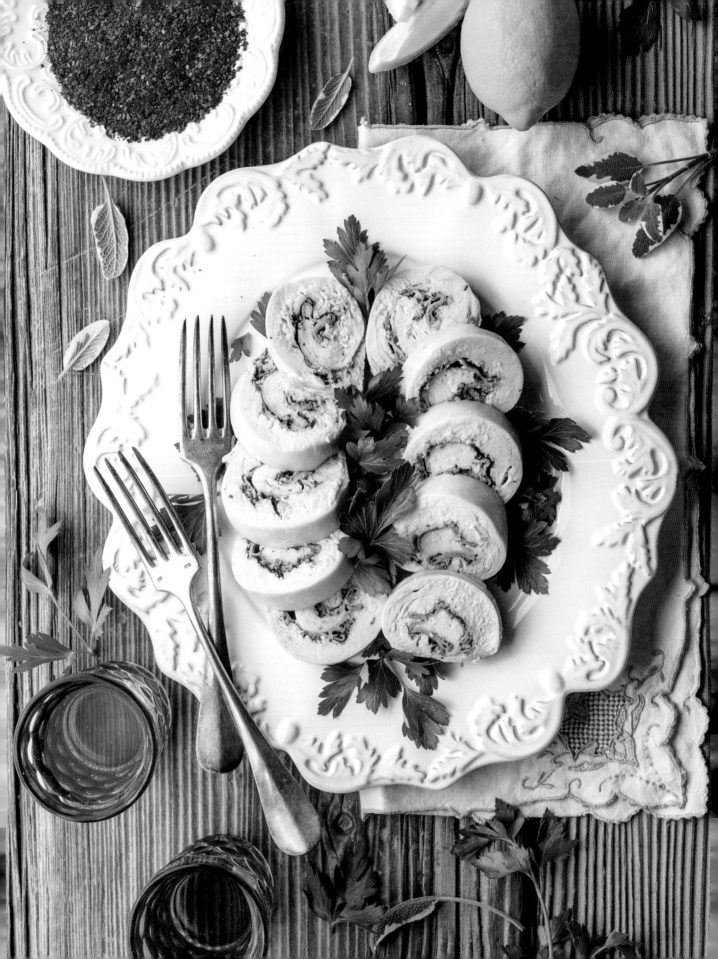

Meal Plans

Notes:

- The following are two sets of meal plans, which provide enough food for two people. The first set comprises four one-week plans designed for three PSMF days per week; the second set includes two one-week plans designed for two PSMF days per week. Both assume that you will be doing regular fat-loss keto on the non-PSMF days.

- The three or two PSMF days can be consecutive or spread out over a week. However, if a day calls for leftovers from the previous PSMF day, it's best to do that day within two days after the meal is made.

- Both sets of plans have been designed for intermittent fasting (IF), with two meals a day eaten within eight hours (ideally within a six-hour window or shorter). Alternatively, you can eat one meal a day if you like.

- The number of servings stated for each recipe corresponds with the number of servings one whole recipe makes. Regardless of how many servings a recipe makes, you should always eat only one serving at each meal.

- Unless otherwise stated, each recipe used in these plans makes two servings. When a recipe makes only one serving, you will need to double it to produce enough food for two people. Likewise, when a recipe makes more than two servings, we either have you eat the leftovers on the following PSMF day or scale the recipe down for two people (please note that not every recipe can be scaled down neatly, but we aim for as little extra food at the end of each week as possible).

x2 *Double the recipe to make 2 servings.*

½ *Halve the recipe to avoid leftovers.*

3 PSMF Days a Week

Week 1

Day 1

Chocolate Breakfast Pudding
84

SNACK:
Egg Salad Sandwiches
Servings: 6
216

Sweet and Sour Pork Chops
Servings: 4 ½
110

END EATING WINDOW

DAY 1 TOTALS

CALORIES	FAT	PROTEIN	CARBS	FIBER
680	26g	93g	13g	2.5g

Day 2

BEGIN EATING WINDOW

Soufflé Omelet with Ham and Chives
Servings: 1 x2
58

LEFTOVER SNACK:
Egg Salad Sandwiches
LEFTOVER

Mediterranean-Style Grilled Swordfish
202

END EATING WINDOW

DAY 2 TOTALS

CALORIES	FAT	PROTEIN	CARBS	FIBER
727	28g	105g	9g	1.3g

Day 3

BEGIN EATING WINDOW

Chocolate Hot Breakfast Cereal
Servings: 1 x2
82

LEFTOVER SNACK:
Egg Salad Sandwiches
LEFTOVER

Baked Chicken Breasts with Ginger Sauce
Servings: 4 ½
152

END EATING WINDOW

DAY 3 TOTALS

CALORIES	FAT	PROTEIN	CARBS	FIBER
768	21g	121g	14g	2.1g

Week 1 Grocery List

PRODUCE:

Chives, 1 bunch

Dill, 1 bunch

Garlic, 8 cloves

Ginger, 3 ounces

Yellow onion, 1 small

MEATS & EGGS:

Chicken breasts, boneless, skinless, 2 (6-ounce)

Egg whites, large, 29

Egg yolks, large, 2

Ham, 95% lean, ½ cup diced

Hard-boiled egg whites, large, 18

Hard-boiled egg yolks, large, 2

Pork chops, bone-in, 2 (5-ounce)

Swordfish fillets, 2 (8-ounce)

PANTRY ITEMS:

Almond milk (or cashew milk), unsweetened, 2½ cups

Beef broth (or chicken broth), ¼ cup

Chicken broth, ¼ cup

Cocoa powder, unsweetened, ⅓ cup

Confectioners'-style erythritol, ½ cup

Dijon mustard (or prepared yellow mustard), ¼ cup

Egg white protein powder, unflavored, 2 tablespoons

Fish stock, ⅓ cup

Tamari, wheat-free, 2 tablespoons

Tomato sauce, 2 tablespoons

STAPLES:

Coconut oil (or lard or tallow)

Coconut vinegar (or apple cider vinegar)

Duck fat spray (or coconut oil spray)

Fine sea salt

Fish sauce

Ground black pepper

Ground cinnamon

Ground coriander

Ground cumin

Liquid stevia

Smoked paprika

Vanilla extract

Week 2

Day 1

Savory Dutch Baby with Lox
68

SNACK:
Snow Cones
240

Basil Shrimp Ceviche
190

END EATING WINDOW

DAY 1 TOTALS

CALORIES	FAT	PROTEIN	CARBS	FIBER
605	14g	109g	6g	1g

Day 2

BEGIN EATING WINDOW

Breakfast Sammie*
Servings: 1 x4
64

SNACK:
Fruity Ice Pops
Servings: 4
241

Grilled Chicken Breasts with Tomato Basil Sauce
138 *Servings: 4*

END EATING WINDOW

DAY 2 TOTALS

CALORIES	FAT	PROTEIN	CARBS	FIBER
642	18g	112g	10g	1.2g

Day 3

BEGIN EATING WINDOW

LEFTOVER Breakfast Sammie

LEFTOVER SNACK:
Fruity Ice Pops

LEFTOVER Grilled Chicken Breasts with Tomato Basil Sauce

END EATING WINDOW

DAY 3 TOTALS

CALORIES	FAT	PROTEIN	CARBS	FIBER
642	18g	112g	10g	1.2g

* Freeze the leftover Breakfast Patties (page 62) to eat later; halve the recipe to have fewer extras.

Week 1 Grocery List

PRODUCE:

Basil, 1 bunch

Dill, 1 bunch

Garlic, 4 cloves

Lime juice, ¾ cup

Red onion, 1 small

MEATS & EGGS:

Chicken breasts, boneless, skinless, 4 (6-ounce)

Egg whites, large, 16

Ground pork, 95% lean, 2 pounds

Ham, 95% lean, 4 slices

Lox (or smoked salmon), 2 ounces

Shrimp, small, 1 pound

PANTRY ITEMS:

Almond milk (or cashew milk), unsweetened, 1⅓ cups

Beef broth, 2¾ cups

Carbonated water, 1 cup

Dried basil leaves, 2 tablespoons

Egg white protein powder, unflavored, ½ cup

Tomato sauce, ½ cup

STAPLES:

Baking powder

Coconut oil

Coconut oil spray

Cream of tartar

Dried rubbed sage

Dried thyme leaves

Duck fat

Duck fat spray

Fine sea salt

Garlic powder

Ground black pepper

Liquid stevia, unflavored and strawberry-flavored

Olive oil, extra-virgin

3 PSMF Days a Week

Week 3

Day 1

BEGIN EATING WINDOW	
88	Orange Creamsicle Smoothie
214	**SNACK:** Meatball Soup *Servings: 8*
146	Thanksgiving Turkey Breast* *Servings: 4*
END EATING WINDOW	

DAY 1 TOTALS

CALORIES	FAT	PROTEIN	CARBS	FIBER
779	17g	141g	5g	1.6g

Day 2

BEGIN EATING WINDOW	
54	Turkey Frittata**
LEFTOVER 214	**SNACK:** Meatball Soup
148	Bourbon Chicken *Servings: 4*
END EATING WINDOW	

DAY 2 TOTALS

CALORIES	FAT	PROTEIN	CARBS	FIBER
642	18g	112g	10g	1.2g

Day 3

BEGIN EATING WINDOW	
60	Steak and Eggs
LEFTOVER	**SNACK:** Meatball Soup
LEFTOVER	Bourbon Chicken
END EATING WINDOW	

DAY 3 TOTALS

CALORIES	FAT	PROTEIN	CARBS	FIBER
742	20g	133g	5g	0.8g

* Use leftover turkey to make the Turkey Frittata on Day 2.
** Use leftover turkey from Day 1.

Week 3 Grocery List

PRODUCE:

Garlic, 2 cloves

Ginger, 1 ounce

Green onions, 1 bunch

Rosemary, 1 bunch

Sage, 1 bunch

Tarragon, 1 bunch

Thyme, 1 bunch

Yellow onion, 1 large

MEATS & EGGS:

Chicken breasts, boneless, skinless, 2 pounds

Egg whites, large, 22

Ground beef, 95% lean, 2 pounds

Turkey breast, boneless, skinless, 1 (2-pound)

Venison (or beef) tenderloin steaks, 2 (4-ounce)

PANTRY ITEMS:

Almond milk (or cashew milk), unsweetened, 1½ cups

Beef broth, 5 cups

Chicken broth, ½ cup

Coconut vinegar (or apple cider vinegar), 1 tablespoon

Confectioners'-style erythritol, ¾ cup

Dijon mustard, 3 tablespoons

Tamari, wheat-free, ⅓ cup

Tomato sauce, ¼ cup

STAPLES:

Coconut oil

Dried rubbed sage

Dried thyme leaves

Duck fat spray

Fine sea salt

Ground black pepper

Liquid stevia, orange-flavored

Onion salt

Orange extract

Red pepper flakes

Week 4

Day 1

BEGIN EATING WINDOW

Apple Dutch Baby
70

SNACK:
Buffalo Chicken Meatballs x2
150

Sorrento Fish
Servings: 4 1/2
192

END EATING WINDOW

DAY 1 TOTALS

CALORIES	FAT	PROTEIN	CARBS	FIBER
674	9g	135g	7g	2g

Day 2

BEGIN EATING WINDOW

Chocolate Breakfast Pudding
84

LEFTOVER SNACK:
Buffalo Chicken Meatballs
150

Saltimbocca-Style Chicken Breasts
Servings: 4
140

END EATING WINDOW

DAY 2 TOTALS

CALORIES	FAT	PROTEIN	CARBS	FIBER
595	11g	113g	9g	4g

Day 3

BEGIN EATING WINDOW

Chocolate Hot Breakfast Cereal
Servings: 1 x2
82

SNACK:
Asian-Style Meatballs*
Servings: 8 1/2
108

LEFTOVER Saltimbocca-Style Chicken Breasts

END EATING WINDOW

DAY 3 TOTALS

CALORIES	FAT	PROTEIN	CARBS	FIBER
792	24g	120g	11g	2.4g

* The leftover meatballs can be eaten on non-PSMF days or frozen for later.

Week 4 Grocery List

PRODUCE:

Celery, 3 stalks

Chives, 1 bunch

Garlic, 7 cloves

Ginger, 1 ounce

Green onions, 1 bunch

Lemon juice, ¼ cup

Mushrooms, button, 2 ounces

Parsley, 1 bunch

Rosemary, 1 bunch

MEATS & EGGS:

Chicken breasts, boneless, skinless, 4 (6-ounce)

Cod fillets (or other white fish fillets), 2 (6-ounce)

Egg whites, large, 28

Ground beef, 95% lean, 1 pound

Ground chicken, extra-lean, 2 pounds

Ham, 95% lean, 4 slices

Hard-boiled egg whites, large, 9

PANTRY ITEMS:

Almond milk (or cashew milk), unsweetened, 3¼ cups

Beef broth, 2 tablespoons

Capers, 1 tablespoon

Cocoa powder, unsweetened, ½ cup

Confectioners'-style erythritol, ½ cup

Egg white protein powder, unflavored, ¼ cup

Hot sauce, 1 cup

Tamari, wheat-free, ¾ teaspoon

Tomato sauce, 1½ teaspoons

STAPLES:

Apple extract

Baking powder

Coconut oil

Coconut oil spray

Dried rubbed sage

Fine sea salt

Ground black pepper

Ground cinnamon

Ground fennel

Liquid stevia

Red pepper flakes

Vanilla extract

2 PSMF Days a Week

Week 1

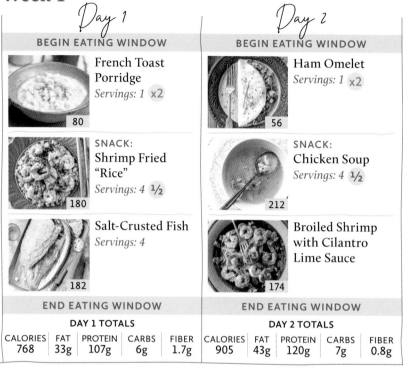

Day 1		*Day 2*	
BEGIN EATING WINDOW		**BEGIN EATING WINDOW**	
French Toast Porridge *Servings: 1* x2	80	Ham Omelet *Servings: 1* x2	56
SNACK: Shrimp Fried "Rice" *Servings: 4* ½	180	SNACK: Chicken Soup *Servings: 4* ½	212
Salt-Crusted Fish *Servings: 4*	182	Broiled Shrimp with Cilantro Lime Sauce	174
END EATING WINDOW		**END EATING WINDOW**	

DAY 1 TOTALS					DAY 2 TOTALS				
CALORIES	FAT	PROTEIN	CARBS	FIBER	CALORIES	FAT	PROTEIN	CARBS	FIBER
768	33g	107g	6g	1.7g	905	43g	120g	7g	0.8g

Week 1 Grocery List

PRODUCE:

Dill, 1 bunch

Garlic, 4 cloves

Jalapeño pepper, 1

Lemons, 2

Limes, 4

Red onion, 1 small

Yellow onion, 1 small

MEATS & EGGS:

Chicken breasts, boneless, skinless, 9 ounces

Egg whites, large, 34

Ham, 95% lean, 4 ounces

Shrimp, large, 8 ounces

Shrimp, medium, 8 ounces

Whole fish, 1 (3-pound)

PANTRY ITEMS:

Almond milk (or cashew milk), unsweetened, 1 ⅓ cups

Beef broth, 1 tablespoon

Capers, 2 tablespoons

Chicken broth, 4¼ cups

Coarse sea salt, 2 cups

Confectioners'-style erythritol, ½ cup

Tamari, wheat-free, 1 teaspoon

STAPLES:

Coconut oil

Fine sea salt

Ground black pepper

Ground cinnamon

Ground cumin

Maple extract

Red pepper flakes

Smoked paprika

Week 2

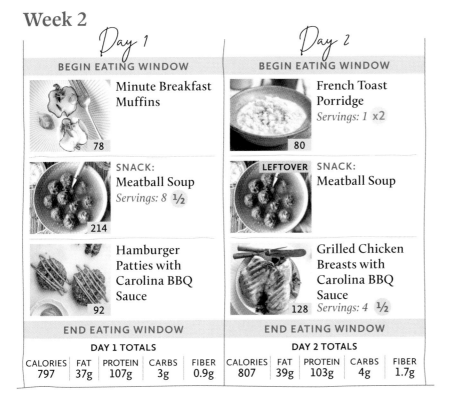

Day 1

BEGIN EATING WINDOW

Minute Breakfast Muffins — 78

SNACK: Meatball Soup — *Servings: 8* ½ — 214

Hamburger Patties with Carolina BBQ Sauce — 92

END EATING WINDOW

DAY 1 TOTALS

CALORIES	FAT	PROTEIN	CARBS	FIBER
797	37g	107g	3g	0.9g

Day 2

BEGIN EATING WINDOW

French Toast Porridge — *Servings: 1* x2 — 80

LEFTOVER SNACK: Meatball Soup

Grilled Chicken Breasts with Carolina BBQ Sauce — 128 — *Servings: 4* ½

END EATING WINDOW

DAY 2 TOTALS

CALORIES	FAT	PROTEIN	CARBS	FIBER
807	39g	103g	4g	1.7g

Week 2 Grocery List

PRODUCE:

Basil, 1 bunch

Garlic, 1 clove

Yellow onion, 1 medium

MEATS & EGGS:

Chicken breasts, boneless, skinless, 2 (6-ounce)

Egg whites, large, 29

Ground beef, 95% lean, 2 pounds

Ham, 95% lean, 6 (4-inch) slices

PANTRY ITEMS:

Almond milk (or cashew milk), unsweetened, 1 ⅓ cups

Beef broth, 3 cups

Coconut vinegar (or apple cider vinegar), ¾ cup

Confectioners'-style erythritol, ½ cup

Prepared yellow mustard, 1 cup

STAPLES:

Cayenne pepper

Chili powder

Coconut oil

Dried thyme leaves

Duck fat

Fine sea salt

Garlic powder

Ground black pepper

Ground cinnamon

Ground white pepper

Liquid smoke

Liquid stevia

Maple extract

Recipe Index

chapter 1 Breakfast

Turkey Frittata

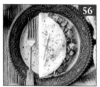
Ham Omelet

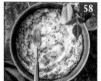
Soufflé Omelet with
Ham and Chives

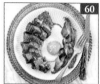
Steak and Eggs

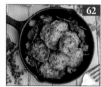
Breakfast Patties

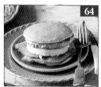
Breakfast Sammie

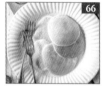
Protein-Sparing
Pancakes

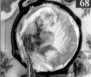
Savory Dutch Baby
with Lox

Apple Dutch Baby

Cinnamon Roll
Waffles

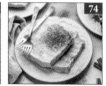
Classic
French Toast

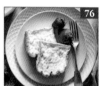
Strawberry Angel
Food French Toast

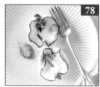
Minute Breakfast
Muffins

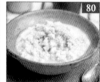
French Toast
Porridge

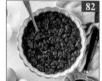
Chocolate Hot
Breakfast Cereal

Chocolate
Breakfast Pudding

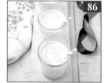
Strawberry Shake

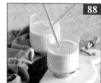
Orange Creamsicle
Smoothie

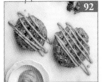
Hamburger Patties
with Mustard

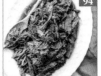
Slow Cooker
Shredded Pork Loin

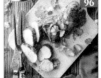
Baked
Pork Tenderloins

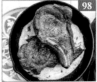
Pork Chops with
Dijon Vinaigrette

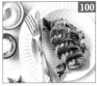
Grilled Filet Mignons with
Truffle Mustard Sauce

BBQ Pork Chops

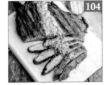
Grilled Flank Steak
with Chimichurri Sauce

BBQ Meatloaf

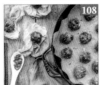
Asian-Style
Meatballs

Sweet and Sour
Pork Chops

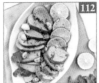
Garlic-Thyme
Pork Tenderloins

BBQ Meatballs

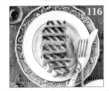
Grilled Pork Chops with
Truffle Mustard Sauce

Poultry

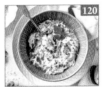
Slow Cooker
Ranch Chicken

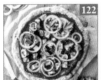
BBQ Chicken
Flatbread

Smoked
Chicken Breasts

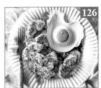
Chicken Strips with
Carolina BBQ Sauce

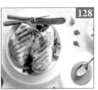
Grilled Chicken Breasts
with Carolina BBQ Sauce

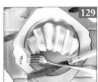
Poached
Chicken Breasts

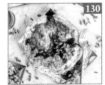
Egg Foo Young

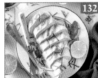
Mojito Chicken

BBQ Grilled
Chicken

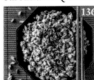
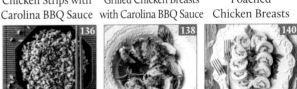
Asian-Inspired
Stir-Fried Turkey

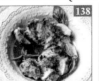
Grilled Chicken Breasts
with Tomato Basil Sauce

Saltimbocca-Style
Chicken Breasts

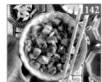
Orange Chicken

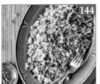
Chicken
Fried "Rice"

Thanksgiving
Turkey Breast

Bourbon Chicken

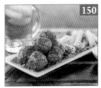
Buffalo Chicken
Meatballs

Baked Chicken
Breasts with
Ginger Sauce

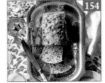
Turkey Meatloaf
with Dijon Sauce

Slow Cooker
Doro Wat

Seafood

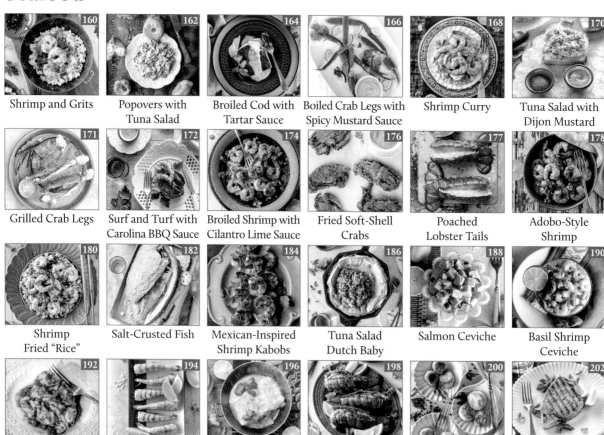

160 — Shrimp and Grits

162 — Popovers with Tuna Salad

164 — Broiled Cod with Tartar Sauce

166 — Boiled Crab Legs with Spicy Mustard Sauce

168 — Shrimp Curry

170 — Tuna Salad with Dijon Mustard

171 — Grilled Crab Legs

172 — Surf and Turf with Carolina BBQ Sauce

174 — Broiled Shrimp with Cilantro Lime Sauce

176 — Fried Soft-Shell Crabs

177 — Poached Lobster Tails

178 — Adobo-Style Shrimp

180 — Shrimp Fried "Rice"

182 — Salt-Crusted Fish

184 — Mexican-Inspired Shrimp Kabobs

186 — Tuna Salad Dutch Baby

188 — Salmon Ceviche

190 — Basil Shrimp Ceviche

192 — Sorrento Fish

194 — Peel-and-Eat Ginger-Lime Shrimp

196 — Halibut with Ginger Sauce

198 — Baked Garlic and Herb Lobster Tails

200 — Broiled Scallops

202 — Mediterranean-Style Grilled Swordfish

204 — Shrimp Scampi

206 — Salmon in Ramen Broth

 chapter 3 # Sides & Snacks

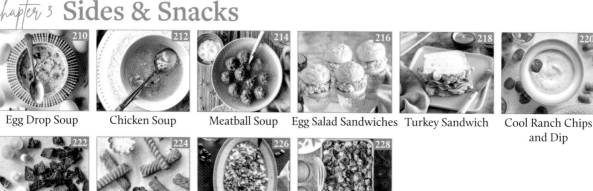

210 — Egg Drop Soup

212 — Chicken Soup

214 — Meatball Soup

216 — Egg Salad Sandwiches

218 — Turkey Sandwich

220 — Cool Ranch Chips and Dip

222 — Venison Jerky

224 — Salmon Jerky

226 — Fried "Rice"

228 — Thanksgiving Stuffing

Desserts & Sweet Treats

chapter 4

232
Strawberry Pavlova

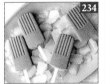
234
Fudge Pops

235
Electrolyte
Ice Pops

236
Orange Creamsicle
Ice Pops

238
Electrolyte
Gummies

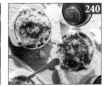
240
Snow Cones

241
Fruity Ice Pops

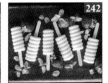
242
Strawberry
Protein Pops

243
Strawberries and
Cream Ice Pops

244
Chocolate
Meringue Cookies

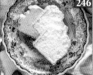
246
Strawberry
Angel Food Cake

248
Vanilla Angel Food
Cupcakes

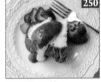
250
Strawberry
Shortcake

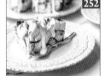
252
Bread Pudding

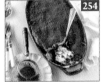
254
Tiramisu

256
Boccone Dolce
Cake

Sauces & Basics

chapter 5

260
Chimichurri Sauce

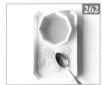
262
Orange Marmalade

264
Spicy BBQ
Vinegar Sauce

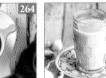
266
Dijon Vinaigrette

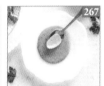
267
Carolina
BBQ Sauce

268
Cilantro Lime Sauce

269
Mayo

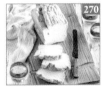
270
Protein-Sparing
Bread

272
Protein-Sparing
Waffle Buns

274
Basil Wraps

Allergen Index

Recipe	Page	🥛	🥜	🌾
Turkey Frittata	54	✓		✓
Ham Omelet	56	✓		✓
Soufflé Omelet with Ham and Chives	58	✓		✓
Steak and Eggs	60	✓		✓
Breakfast Patties	62	✓	✓	✓
Breakfast Sammie	64	✓		✓
Protein-Sparing Pancakes	66	✓		✓
Savory Dutch Baby with Lox	68	✓		✓
Apple Dutch Baby	70	✓		
Cinnamon Roll Waffles	72	✓		✓
Classic French Toast	74	✓		✓
Strawberry Angel Food French Toast	76	✓		✓
Minute Breakfast Muffins	78	✓		✓
French Toast Porridge	80	✓		
Chocolate Hot Breakfast Cereal	82	✓		
Chocolate Breakfast Pudding	84	✓		
Strawberry Shake	86	✓	✓	
Orange Creamsicle Smoothie	88	✓		
Hamburger Patties with Mustard	92	✓	✓	✓
Slow Cooker Shredded Pork Loin	94	✓	✓	✓
Baked Pork Tenderloins	96	✓	✓	✓
Pork Chops with Dijon Vinaigrette	98	✓	✓	✓
Grilled Filet Mignons with Truffle Mustard Sauce	100	✓	✓	✓
BBQ Pork Chops	102	✓	✓	✓
Grilled Flank Steak with Chimichurri Sauce	104	✓	✓	✓
BBQ Meatloaf	106	✓		✓
Asian-Style Meatballs	108	✓		✓
Sweet and Sour Pork Chops	110	✓	✓	✓
Garlic-Thyme Pork Tenderloins	112	✓	✓	✓
BBQ Meatballs	114	✓		✓
Grilled Pork Chops with Truffle Mustard Sauce	116	✓	✓	✓
Slow Cooker Ranch Chicken	120	✓	✓	✓
BBQ Chicken Flatbread	122	✓		✓
Smoked Chicken Breasts	124	✓	✓	✓
Chicken Strips with Carolina BBQ Sauce	126	✓	✓	✓
Grilled Chicken Breasts with Carolina BBQ Sauce	128	✓	✓	✓
Poached Chicken Breasts	129	✓	✓	✓
Egg Foo Young	130	✓		✓
Mojito Chicken	132	✓	✓	✓
BBQ Grilled Chicken	134	✓	✓	✓
Asian-Inspired Stir-Fried Turkey	136	✓	✓	✓
Grilled Chicken Breasts with Tomato Basil Sauce	138	✓	✓	✓
Saltimbocca-Style Chicken Breasts	140	✓	✓	✓
Orange Chicken	142	✓	✓	✓
Chicken Fried "Rice"	144	✓		✓
Thanksgiving Turkey Breast	146	✓	✓	✓
Bourbon Chicken	148	✓		✓
Buffalo Chicken Meatballs	150	✓		✓
Baked Chicken Breasts with Ginger Sauce	152	✓	✓	✓
Turkey Meatloaf with Dijon Sauce	154	✓		✓
Slow Cooker Doro Wat	156	✓		✓
Shrimp and Grits	160	✓		✓
Popovers with Tuna Salad	162	✓		
Broiled Cod with Tartar Sauce	164	✓		✓

Recipe	Page	🥛⃠	🥚⃠	🥜⃠
Boiled Crab Legs with Spicy Mustard Sauce	166	✓		✓
Shrimp Curry	168	✓	✓	✓
Tuna Salad with Dijon Mustard	170	✓		✓
Grilled Crab Legs	171	✓	✓	✓
Surf and Turf with Carolina BBQ Sauce	172	✓	✓	✓
Broiled Shrimp with Cilantro Lime Sauce	174	✓	✓	✓
Fried Soft-Shell Crabs	176	✓		✓
Poached Lobster Tails	177	✓	✓	✓
Adobo-Style Shrimp	178	✓	✓	✓
Shrimp Fried "Rice"	180	✓		✓
Salt-Crusted Fish	182	✓		✓
Mexican-Inspired Shrimp Kabobs	184	✓	✓	✓
Tuna Salad Dutch Baby	186	✓		✓
Salmon Ceviche	188	✓	✓	✓
Basil Shrimp Ceviche	190	✓	✓	✓
Shrimp Scampi	204	✓	✓	✓
Sorrento Fish	192	✓	✓	✓
Peel-and-Eat Ginger-Lime Shrimp	194	✓	✓	✓
Halibut with Ginger Sauce	196	✓	✓	✓
Baked Garlic and Herb Lobster Tails	198	✓	✓	✓
Broiled Scallops	200	✓	✓	✓
Mediterranean-Style Grilled Swordfish	202	✓	✓	✓
Salmon in Ramen Broth	206	✓	✓	✓
Egg Drop Soup	210	✓		✓
Chicken Soup	212	✓	✓	✓
Meatball Soup	214	✓		✓
Egg Salad Sandwiches	216	✓		✓
Turkey Sandwich	218	✓		✓
Cool Ranch Chips and Dip	220	✓		✓
Venison Jerky	222	✓	✓	✓
Salmon Jerky	224	✓	✓	✓
Fried "Rice"	226	✓		✓
Thanksgiving Stuffing	228	✓		✓
Strawberry Pavlova	232	✓		✓
Fudge Pops	234	✓		
Electrolyte Ice Pops	235	✓	✓	✓
Orange Creamsicle Ice Pops	236	✓		
Electrolyte Gummies	238	✓	✓	✓
Snow Cones	240	✓	✓	✓
Fruity Ice Pops	241	✓	✓	✓
Strawberry Protein Pops	242	✓	✓	
Strawberries and Cream Ice Pops	243	✓		
Chocolate Meringue Cookies	244	✓		✓
Strawberry Angel Food Cake	246	✓		✓
Vanilla Angel Food Cupcakes	248	✓		✓
Strawberry Shortcake	250	✓		
Bread Pudding	252	✓		
Tiramisu	254	✓		
Boccone Dolce Cake	256	✓		
Chimichurri Sauce	260	✓	✓	✓
Orange Marmalade	262	✓	✓	✓
Spicy BBQ Vinegar Sauce	264	✓	✓	✓
Dijon Vinaigrette	266	✓	✓	✓
Carolina BBQ Sauce	267	✓	✓	✓
Cilantro Lime Sauce	268	✓	✓	✓
Mayo	269	✓		✓
Protein-Sparing Bread	270	✓		✓
Protein-Sparing Waffle Buns	272	✓		✓
Basil Wraps	274	✓		✓

General Index

A

acetyl coenzyme A (acetyl-CoA), 28–29

acylation-stimulating protein (ASP), 11–13

adenosine triphosphate (ATP), 28–29

Adobo-Style Shrimp recipe, 178–179

alcohol, oxidative priority and, 25

almond milk

    Apple Dutch Baby, 70–71

    Banana Breakfast Pudding, 84

    Black Forest Breakfast Pudding, 84

    Boccone Dolce Cake, 256–257

    Bread Pudding, 252–253

    Butterscotch Breakfast Pudding, 84

    Chocolate Breakfast Pudding, 84–85

    Chocolate Hot Breakfast Cereal, 82–83

    French Toast Breakfast Pudding, 84

    French Toast Porridge, 80–81

    French Vanilla Breakfast Pudding, 84

    Fudge Pops, 234

    Key Lime Breakfast Pudding, 84

    Lemon Breakfast Pudding, 84

    Orange Creamsicle Ice Pops, 236–237

    Orange Creamsicle Smoothie, 88–89

    Popovers with Tuna Salad, 162–163

    Shrimp and Grits, 160–161

    Strawberry and Cream Ice Pops, 243

    Strawberry Protein Pops, 242

    Strawberry Shake, 86–87

    Strawberry Shortcake, 250–251

    Tiramisu, 254–255

amino acids, 9, 34

animal proteins, nutrients in, 33

Apple Dutch Baby recipe, 70–71

apples, nutrients in, 32

Asian-Inspired Stir-Fried Turkey recipe, 136–137

Asian-Style Meatballs recipe, 108–109

autophagy, 17–19

B

Baked Chicken Breasts with Ginger Sauce recipe, 152–153

Baked Garlic and Herb Lobster Tails recipe, 198–199

Baked Pork Tenderloins recipe, 96–97

Banana Breakfast Pudding recipe, 84

basal metabolic rate (BMR), 9, 37–38

basil

    Basil Shrimp Ceviche, 190–191

    Basil Wraps, 274–275

    Grilled Chicken Breasts with Tomato Basil Sauce, 138–139

    Minute Breakfast Muffins, 78–79

    Shrimp Scampi, 204–205

Basil Shrimp Ceviche recipe, 190–191

Basil Wraps recipe, 274–275

bay leaves

    Poached Chicken Breasts, 129

BBQ Chicken Flatbread recipe, 122–123

BBQ Grilled Chicken recipe, 134–135

    BBQ Chicken Flatbread, 122–123

BBQ Meatballs recipe, 114–115

BBQ Meatloaf recipe, 106–107

BBQ Pork Chops recipe, 102–103

BBQ Sauce recipe

    BBQ Chicken Flatbread, 122–123

    BBQ Grilled Chicken, 134–135

    BBQ Meatloaf, 106–107

    Smoked Chicken Breasts, 124–125

beef

    Asian-Style Meatballs, 108–109

    BBQ Meatballs, 114–115

    BBQ Meatloaf, 106–107

    Grilled Filet Mignons with Truffle Mustard Sauce, 100–101

    Grilled Flank Steak with Chimichurri Sauce, 104–105

    Hamburger Patties with Mustard, 92–93

    Meatball Soup, 214–215

    for muscle building, 34

    nutrients in, 13, 14, 32, 33

    P/E ratio of, 45

    Steak and Eggs, 60–61

    Surf and Turf with Carolina BBQ Sauce, 172–173

    Venison Jerky, 222–223

beef broth

    Baked Chicken Breasts with Ginger Sauce, 152–153

    BBQ Meatballs, 114–115

    Chicken Fried "Rice," 144–145

    Cool Ranch Chips and Dip, 220–221

    Fried "Rice," 226–227

    Grilled Chicken Breasts with Tomato Basil Sauce, 138–139

    Halibut with Ginger Sauce, 196–197

    Mayo, 269

    Meatball Soup, 214–215

    Mediterranean-Style Grilled Swordfish, 202–203

    Savory Dutch Baby with Lox, 68–69

    Shrimp Fried "Rice," 180–181

    Sorrento Fish, 192–193

    Tuna Salad Dutch Baby, 186–187

    Turkey Meatloaf with Dijon Sauce, 154–155

beef liver, nutrients in, 32, 33

berbere

    Slow Cooker Doro Wat, 156–157

beta-oxidation, 28

Black Forest Breakfast Pudding recipe, 84

black truffle

    Grilled Filet Mignons with Truffle Mustard Sauce, 100–101

Blackburn, George, 7

BLC2 genes, 18

blueberries, nutrients in, 32

blue-blocking glasses, sleep and, 49

Boccone Dolce Cake recipe, 256–257

Boiled Crab Legs with Spicy Mustard Sauce recipe, 166–167

Bourbon Chicken recipe, 148–149

bowel movements, 19

Bread Pudding recipe, 252–253

Breakfast Patties recipe, 62–63

    Breakfast Sammie, 64–65

Breakfast Sammie recipe, 64–65

broccoli, for muscle building, 34

Broiled Cod with Tartar Sauce recipe, 164–165

Broiled Scallops recipe, 200–201

Broiled Shrimp with Cilantro Lime Sauce recipe, 174–175

Buffalo Chicken Meatballs recipe, 150–151

bulletproof coffee, 26

butter coffee, nutrients in, 13–14

Butterscotch Breakfast Pudding recipe, 84

C

cabbage

    Egg Foo Young, 130–131

caffeinated drinks, PSMF and, 48

cakes

    Boccone Dolce Cake, 256–257

    Classic Angel Food Cake, 246–247

    Strawberry Angel Food Cake, 246–247

    Strawberry Shortcake, 250–251

    Vanilla Angel Food Cupcakes, 248–249

calories

    about, 10

    fat, 13–15

    miscalculation of intake, 36

capers

    Salt-Crusted Fish, 182–183

    Sorrento Fish, 192–193

carbohydrates, oxidative priority and, 26

carbonated water

    Fruity Ice Pops, 241

Carolina BBQ Sauce recipe, 267

    Chicken Strips with Carolina BBQ Sauce, 126–127

    Fried Soft-Shell Crab, 176

    Grilled Chicken Breasts with Carolina BBQ Sauce, 128

    Hamburger Patties with Mustard, 92–93

    Poached Lobster Tails, 177

    Surf and Turf with Carolina BBQ Sauce, 172–173

cashew milk

    Apple Dutch Baby, 70–71

    Banana Breakfast Pudding, 84

    Black Forest Breakfast Pudding, 84

cashew milk (*continued*)

Bread Pudding, 252–253

Butterscotch Breakfast Pudding, 84

Chocolate Breakfast Pudding, 84–85

Chocolate Hot Breakfast Cereal, 82–83

French Toast Breakfast Pudding, 84

French Toast Porridge, 80–81

French Vanilla Breakfast Pudding, 84

Fudge Pops, 234

Key Lime Breakfast Pudding, 84

Lemon Breakfast Pudding, 84

Orange Creamsicle Ice Pops, 236–237

Orange Creamsicle Smoothie, 88–89

Popovers with Tuna Salad, 162–163

Shrimp and Grits, 160–161

Strawberry and Cream Ice Pops, 243

Strawberry Protein Pops, 242

Strawberry Shake, 86–87

Strawberry Shortcake, 250–251

Tiramisu, 254–255

celery

Buffalo Chicken Meatballs, 150–151

Thanksgiving Stuffing, 228–229

cellular respiration, 26–31

chicken

Asian-Inspired Stir-Fried Turkey, 136–137

Baked Chicken Breasts with Ginger Sauce, 152–153

Basil Wraps, 274–275

BBQ Grilled Chicken, 134–135

Bourbon Chicken, 148–149

Buffalo Chicken Meatballs, 150–151

Chicken Fried "Rice," 144–145

Chicken Soup, 212–213

Chicken Strips with Carolina BBQ Sauce, 126–127

Cool Ranch Chips and Dip, 220–221

Egg Foo Young, 130–131

Grilled Chicken Breasts with Carolina BBQ Sauce, 128

Grilled Chicken Breasts with Tomato Basil Sauce, 138–139

Mojito Chicken, 132–133

nutrients in, 33

Orange Chicken, 142–143

Poached Chicken Breasts, 129

Saltimbocca-Style Chicken Breasts, 140–141

Slow Cooker Doro Wat, 156–157

Slow Cooker Ranch Chicken, 120–121

Smoked Chicken Breasts, 124–125

chicken broth

Baked Chicken Breasts with Ginger Sauce, 152–153

BBQ Meatballs, 114–115

Bourbon Chicken, 148–149

Chicken Soup, 212–213

Cilantro Lime Sauce, 268

Egg Drop Soup, 210–211

Egg Foo Young, 130–131

Halibut with Ginger Sauce, 196–197

Poached Chicken Breasts, 129

Salmon in Ramen Broth, 206–207

Shrimp Curry, 168–169

Shrimp Scampi, 204–205

Slow Cooker Doro Wat, 156–157

Slow Cooker Ranch Chicken, 120–121

Slow Cooker Shredded Pork Loin, 94–95

Sweet and Sour Pork Chops, 110–111

Thanksgiving Stuffing, 228–229

Turkey Meatloaf with Dijon Sauce, 154–155

Chicken Fried "Rice" recipe, 144–145

Chicken Soup recipe, 212–213

Chicken Strips with Carolina BBQ Sauce recipe, 126–127

Chimichurri Sauce recipe, 260–261

Grilled Flank Steak with Chimichurri Sauce, 104–105

chives

Saltimbocca-Style Chicken Breasts, 140–141

Souffle Omelet with Ham and Chives, 58–59

chocolate

Boccone Dolce Cake, 256–257

Chocolate Breakfast Pudding recipe, 84–85

Chocolate Hot Breakfast Cereal recipe, 82–83

Chocolate Meringue Cookies recipe, 244–245

chylomicrons, 10

cilantro

Adobo-Style Shrimp, 178–179

Broiled Shrimp with Cilantro Lime Sauce, 174–175

Chicken Soup, 212–213

Chimichurri Sauce, 260–261

Cilantro Lime Sauce, 268

Halibut with Ginger Sauce, 196–197

Salmon Ceviche, 188–189

Shrimp and Grits, 160–161

Shrimp Curry, 168–169

Slow Cooker Doro Wat, 156–157

Cilantro Lime Sauce recipe, 268

Broiled Shrimp with Cilantro Lime Sauce, 174–175

cinnamon

Cinnamon Protein-Sparing Bread, 270–271

Cinnamon Roll Waffles, 72–73

Classic French Toast, 74–75

French Toast Breakfast Pudding, 84

Cinnamon Protein-Sparing Bread recipe, 270–271

Classic French Toast, 74–75

Cinnamon Roll Waffles recipe, 72–73

citric acid cycle, 26–31

Classic Angel Food Cake recipe, 246–247

Classic French Toast recipe, 74–75

cocoa powder

Black Forest Breakfast Pudding, 84

Boccone Dolce Cake, 256–257

Chocolate Breakfast Pudding, 84–85

Chocolate Hot Breakfast Cereal, 82–83

Chocolate Meringue Cookies, 244–245

Fudge Pops, 234

Tiramisu, 254–255

cod

Broiled Cod with Tartar Sauce, 164–165

Sorrento Fish, 192–193

coffee

Tiramisu, 254–255

Cool Ranch Chips and Dip recipe, 220–221

crab

Boiled Crab Legs with Spicy Mustard Sauce, 166–167

Fried Soft-Shell Crab, 176

Grilled Crab Legs, 171

curry paste

Shrimp Curry, 168–169

D

dietary fat, fat fasting and, 9–13

Dijon mustard

Boiled Crab Legs with Spicy Mustard Sauce, 166–167

Dijon Vinaigrette, 266

Egg Salad Sandwiches, 216–217

Grilled Filet Mignons with Truffle Mustard Sauce, 100–101

Popovers with Tuna Salad, 162–163

Thanksgiving Turkey Breast, 146–147

Tuna Salad Dutch Baby, 186–187

Tuna Salad with Dijon Mustard, 170

Turkey Meatloaf with Dijon Sauce, 154–155

Turkey Sandwich, 218–219

Dijon Vinaigrette recipe, 266

Poached Lobster Tails, 177

Pork Chops with Dijon Vinaigrette, 98–99

dill

Egg Salad Sandwiches, 216–217

Salt-Crusted Fish, 182–183

Savory Dutch Baby with Lox, 68–69

dill pickle juice

Broiled Cod with Tartar Sauce, 164–165

dill pickles

Broiled Cod with Tartar Sauce, 164–165

E

Egg Drop Soup recipe, 210–211

egg fasting, 16

Egg Foo Young recipe, 130–131

Egg Salad Sandwiches recipe, 216–217

eggs

Apple Dutch Baby, 70–71

Asian-Style Meatballs, 108–109

Banana Breakfast Pudding, 84

Basil Wraps, 274–275

BBQ Chicken Flatbread, 122–123

BBQ Meatballs, 114–115

BBQ Meatloaf, 106–107

Black Forest Breakfast Pudding, 84

Boccone Dolce Cake, 256–257

Bread Pudding, 252–253

Breakfast Sammie, 64–65

Buffalo Chicken Meatballs, 150–151

Butterscotch Breakfast Pudding, 84

Chicken Fried "Rice," 144–145

Chocolate Breakfast Pudding, 84–85

Chocolate Hot Breakfast Cereal, 82–83

Chocolate Meringue Cookies, 244–245

Cinnamon Protein-Sparing Bread, 270–271

eggs *(continued)*

Cinnamon Roll Waffles, 72–73

Classic Angel Food Cake, 246–247

Classic French Toast, 74–75

Cool Ranch Chips and Dip, 220–221

Egg Drop Soup, 210–211

egg fasting, 16

Egg Foo Young, 130–131

Egg Salad Sandwiches, 216–217

French Toast Breakfast Pudding, 84

French Toast Porridge, 80–81

French Vanilla Breakfast Pudding, 84

Fried "Rice," 226–227

Fried Soft-Shell Crab, 176

Fudge Pops, 234

Ham Omelet, 56–57

Key Lime Breakfast Pudding, 84

Lemon Breakfast Pudding, 84

Mayo, 269

Meatball Soup, 214–215

Minute Breakfast Muffins, 78–79

nutrients in, 13, 14, 33

Orange Creamsicle Ice Pops, 236–237

Orange Creamsicle Smoothie, 88–89

P/E ratio of, 43

Popovers with Tuna Salad, 162–163

Protein-Sparing Bread, 270–271

Protein-Sparing Pancakes, 66–67

Protein-Sparing Waffle Buns, 272–273

Salt-Crusted Fish, 182–183

Savory Dutch Baby with Lox, 68–69

Shrimp and Grits, 160–161

Shrimp Fried "Rice," 180–181

Slow Cooker Doro Wat, 156–157

Souffle Omelet with Ham and Chives, 58–59

Steak and Eggs, 60–61

Strawberry and Cream Ice Pops, 243

Strawberry Angel Food Cake, 246–247

Strawberry Angel Food French Toast, 76–77

Strawberry Pavlova, 232–233

Strawberry Shortcake, 250–251

Thanksgiving Stuffing, 228–229

Tiramisu, 254–255

Tuna Salad Dutch Baby, 186–187

Turkey Frittata, 54–55

Turkey Meatloaf with Dijon Sauce, 154–155

Vanilla Angel Food Cupcakes, 248–249

electrolyte drink

Electrolyte Gummies, 238–239

Electrolyte Ice Pops, 235

Fruity Ice Pops, 241

Snow Cones, 240

Electrolyte Gummies recipe, 238–239

Electrolyte Ice Pops recipe, 235

Emmerich, Craig, *Keto,* 9

Emmerich, Maria

The 30-Day Ketogenic Cleanse, 40

blog, 40

Keto, 9

Epsom salt bath, sleep and, 49

erythritol

Apple Dutch Baby, 70–71

Banana Breakfast Pudding, 84

Black Forest Breakfast Pudding, 84

Boccone Dolce Cake, 256–257

Bourbon Chicken, 148–149

Bread Pudding, 252–253

Butterscotch Breakfast Pudding, 84

Chocolate Breakfast Pudding, 84–85

Chocolate Meringue Cookies, 244–245

Classic Angel Food Cake, 246–247

French Toast Breakfast Pudding, 84

French Toast Porridge, 80–81

French Vanilla Breakfast Pudding, 84

Fudge Pops, 234

Key Lime Breakfast Pudding, 84

Lemon Breakfast Pudding, 84

Orange Creamsicle Ice Pops, 236–237

Orange Creamsicle Smoothie, 88–89

Orange Marmalade, 262–263

Spicy BBQ Vinegar Sauce, 264–265

Strawberry and Cream Ice Pops, 243

Strawberry Angel Food Cake, 246–247

Strawberry Pavlova, 232–233

Strawberry Shortcake, 250–251

Sweet and Sour Pork Chops, 110–111

Tiramisu, 254–255

Vanilla Angel Food Cupcakes, 248–249

espresso

    Tiramisu, 254–255

essential oils, 49

exercise, PSMF and, 48

exogenous ketones, oxidative priority and, 26

extended fasting, 17–19, 39

F

fasting

    protein-sparing modified fasting (PSMF), 7

    types, 8–23

fat calories

    about, 13–15

    oxidative priority and, 26

fat fasting, 8–15

fat loss, 9–13

fat threshold, 12–13

fatty acid metabolism, 28

fennel

    Saltimbocca-Style Chicken Breasts, 140–141

fish and seafood

    Adobo-Style Shrimp, 178–179

    Baked Garlic and Herb Lobster Tails, 198–199

    Basil Shrimp Ceviche, 190–191

    Boiled Crab Legs with Spicy Mustard Sauce, 166–167

    Broiled Cod with Tartar Sauce, 164–165

    Broiled Scallops, 200–201

    Broiled Shrimp with Cilantro Lime Sauce, 174–175

    Fried Soft-Shell Crab, 176

    Grilled Crab Legs, 171

    Halibut with Ginger Sauce, 196–197

    Mediterranean-Style Grilled Swordfish, 202–203

    Mexican-Inspired Shrimp Kabobs, 184–185

    P/E ratio of, 47

    Peel-and-Eat Ginger-Lime Shrimp, 194–195

    Poached Lobster Tails, 177

    Popovers with Tuna Salad, 162–163

    Salmon Ceviche, 188–189

    Salmon in Ramen Broth, 206–207

    Salmon Jerky, 224–225

    Salt-Crusted Fish, 182–183

    Savory Dutch Baby with Lox, 68–69

    Shrimp and Grits, 160–161

    Shrimp Curry, 168–169

    Shrimp Fried "Rice," 180–181

    Shrimp Scampi, 204–205

    Sorrento Fish, 192–193

    Surf and Turf with Carolina BBQ Sauce, 172–173

    Tuna Salad Dutch Baby, 186–187

    Tuna Salad with Dijon Mustard, 170

fish sauce

    Adobo-Style Shrimp, 178–179

    Baked Chicken Breasts with Ginger Sauce, 152–153

    Egg Drop Soup, 210–211

    Halibut with Ginger Sauce, 196–197

    Mayo, 269

    Meatball Soup, 214–215

fish stock

    Mediterranean-Style Grilled Swordfish, 202–203

free fatty acids (FFA), 28–30

free radical damage, 20

French Toast Breakfast Pudding recipe, 84

French Toast Porridge recipe, 80–81

French Vanilla Breakfast Pudding recipe, 84

    Cinnamon Roll Waffles, 72–73

Fried "Rice" recipe, 226–227

    Adobo-Style Shrimp, 178–179

    Asian-Style Meatballs, 108–109

    Bourbon Chicken, 148–149

    Orange Chicken, 142–143

    Shrimp Curry, 168–169

Fried Soft-Shell Crab recipe, 176

Fruity Ice Pops recipe, 241

Fudge Pops recipe, 234

G

garam masala

    Shrimp Curry, 168–169

garlic

    Adobo-Style Shrimp, 178–179

    Asian-Inspired Stir-Fried Turkey, 136–137

    Asian-Style Meatballs, 108–109

    Baked Chicken Breasts with Ginger Sauce, 152–153

    Baked Garlic and Herb Lobster Tails, 198–199

    Baked Pork Tenderloins, 96–97

    Basil Shrimp Ceviche, 190–191

    BBQ Meatballs, 114–115

    Bourbon Chicken, 148–149

    Breakfast Patties, 62–63

    Broiled Shrimp with Cilantro Lime Sauce, 174–175

    Chicken Fried "Rice," 144–145

    Chicken Soup, 212–213

    Chimichurri Sauce, 260–261

    Cilantro Lime Sauce, 268

    Dijon Vinaigrette, 266

    Egg Foo Young, 130–131

garlic (continued)

Fried "Rice," 226–227

Garlic Thyme Pork Tenderloins, 112–113

Grilled Chicken Breasts with Tomato Basil Sauce, 138–139

Grilled Flank Steak with Chimichurri Sauce, 104–105

Halibut with Ginger Sauce, 196–197

Meatball Soup, 214–215

Mediterranean-Style Grilled Swordfish, 202–203

Mojito Chicken, 132–133

Orange Chicken, 142–143

Poached Chicken Breasts, 129

Salmon Ceviche, 188–189

Salmon in Ramen Broth, 206–207

Salmon Jerky, 224–225

Saltimbocca-Style Chicken Breasts, 140–141

Shrimp Curry, 168–169

Shrimp Fried "Rice," 180–181

Shrimp Scampi, 204–205

Slow Cooker Doro Wat, 156–157

Slow Cooker Shredded Pork Loin, 94–95

Sorrento Fish, 192–193

Sweet and Sour Pork Chops, 110–111

Turkey Meatloaf with Dijon Sauce, 154–155

Venison Jerky, 222–223

Garlic Thyme Pork Tenderloins recipe, 112–113

gelatin

Electrolyte Gummies, 238–239

Orange Marmalade, 262–263

ginger

Asian-Inspired Stir-Fried Turkey, 136–137

Asian-Style Meatballs, 108–109

Baked Chicken Breasts with Ginger Sauce, 152–153

Baked Pork Tenderloins, 96–97

Bourbon Chicken, 148–149

Egg Drop Soup, 210–211

Egg Foo Young, 130–131

Halibut with Ginger Sauce, 196–197

Orange Chicken, 142–143

Peel-and-Eat Ginger-Lime Shrimp, 194–195

Salmon in Ramen Broth, 206–207

Salmon Jerky, 224–225

Shrimp Curry, 168–169

Sweet and Sour Pork Chops, 110–111

Venison Jerky, 222–223

goat, P/E ratio of, 44

green onions

Asian-Inspired Stir-Fried Turkey, 136–137

Asian-Style Meatballs, 108–109

Bourbon Chicken, 148–149

Chicken Fried "Rice," 144–145

Egg Drop Soup, 210–211

Egg Foo Young, 130–131

Fried "Rice," 226–227

Orange Chicken, 142–143

Salmon in Ramen Broth, 206–207

Shrimp Curry, 168–169

Shrimp Fried "Rice," 180–181

Sweet and Sour Pork Chops, 110–111

Tuna Salad Dutch Baby, 186–187

Grilled Chicken Breasts with Carolina BBQ Sauce recipe, 128

Grilled Chicken Breasts with Tomato Basil Sauce recipe, 138–139

Grilled Crab Legs recipe, 171

Grilled Filet Mignons with Truffle Mustard Sauce recipe, 100–101

Grilled Flank Steak with Chimichurri Sauce recipe, 104–105

Grilled Pork Chops with Truffle Mustard Sauce recipe, 116–117

H

Halibut with Ginger Sauce recipe, 196–197

ham

Breakfast Sammie, 64–65

Cool Ranch Chips and Dip, 220–221

Ham Omelet, 56–57

Minute Breakfast Muffins, 78–79

Saltimbocca-Style Chicken Breasts, 140–141

Souffle Omelet with Ham and Chives, 58–59

Ham Omelet recipe, 56–57

Hamburger Patties with Mustard recipe, 92–93

horseradish

Boiled Crab Legs with Spicy Mustard Sauce, 166–167

hot sauce

Boiled Crab Legs with Spicy Mustard Sauce, 166–167

Buffalo Chicken Meatballs, 150–151

Egg Foo Young, 130–131

Spicy BBQ Vinegar Sauce, 264–265

I

inflammation, 20

insulin, 9, 11–13, 20

intermittent fasting, 20–21

J–K

jalapeño peppers

    Cilantro Lime Sauce, 268

kale, nutrients in, 32

Keto (Emmerich and Emmerich), 9

Key Lime Breakfast Pudding
   recipe, 84

Krebs cycle, 26–31

L

lamb, P/E ratio of, 44

lemon

    Broiled Cod with Tartar
      Sauce, 164–165

Lemon Breakfast Pudding recipe,
   84

lemon juice

    Baked Garlic and Herb
      Lobster Tails, 198–199

    Boiled Crab Legs with Spicy
      Mustard Sauce, 166–167

    Broiled Shrimp with Cilantro
      Lime Sauce, 174–175

    Dijon Vinaigrette, 266

    Mediterranean-Style Grilled
      Swordfish, 202–203

    Saltimbocca-Style Chicken
      Breasts, 140–141

    Sorrento Fish, 192–193

    Turkey Meatloaf with Dijon
      Sauce, 154–155

lemons

    Chicken Strips with Carolina
      BBQ Sauce, 126–127

Mediterranean-Style Grilled
   Swordfish, 202–203

Salt-Crusted Fish, 182–183

leptin, 20

lime juice

    Adobo-Style Shrimp, 178–179

    Baked Chicken Breasts with
      Ginger Sauce, 152–153

    Baked Pork Tenderloins,
      96–97

    Basil Shrimp Ceviche, 190–191

    Boiled Crab Legs with Spicy
      Mustard Sauce, 166–167

    Broiled Shrimp with Cilantro
      Lime Sauce, 174–175

    Cilantro Lime Sauce, 268

    Grilled Flank Steak with
      Chimichurri Sauce, 104–105

    Halibut with Ginger Sauce,
      196–197

    Mojito Chicken, 132–133

    Peel-and-Eat Ginger-Lime
      Shrimp, 194–195

    Salmon Ceviche, 188–189

    Salmon Jerky, 224–225

    Shrimp Curry, 168–169

    Venison Jerky, 222–223

limes

    Boiled Crab Legs with Spicy
      Mustard Sauce, 166–167

    Grilled Flank Steak with
      Chimichurri Sauce, 104–105

    Halibut with Ginger Sauce,
      196–197

    Mojito Chicken, 132–133

    Peel-and-Eat Ginger-Lime
      Shrimp, 194–195

    Shrimp Curry, 168–169

lipolysis, 28

liver (beef), nutrients in, 32, 33

lobster

    Baked Garlic and Herb
      Lobster Tails, 198–199

    Poached Lobster Tails, 177

lox

    Savory Dutch Baby with Lox,
      68–69

M

magnesium, sleep and, 49

Mayo recipe, 269

    Boiled Crab Legs with Spicy
      Mustard Sauce, 166–167

    Broiled Cod with Tartar
      Sauce, 164–165

    Popovers with Tuna Salad,
      162–163

    Tuna Salad with Dijon
      Mustard, 170

MCT oil, 14

meal plans, 277–283

Meatball Soup recipe, 214–215

Mediterranean-Style Grilled
   Swordfish recipe, 202–203

metabolic adaptation, 37–38

Mexican-Inspired Shrimp Kabobs
   recipe, 184–185

mint

    Mojito Chicken, 132–133

Minute Breakfast Muffins recipe,
   78–79

Mojito Chicken recipe, 132–133

muscle, protein requirements for
   building, 34

muscle protein synthesis (mTOR),
   34

mushrooms

    Asian-Style Meatballs,
      108–109

    BBQ Meatloaf, 106–107

    Egg Drop Soup, 210–211

    Egg Foo Young, 130–131

    Thanksgiving Stuffing,
      228–229

mushrooms (continued)

    Turkey Meatloaf with Dijon Sauce, 154–155

N

Naiman, Ted, *The P:E Diet*, 42

nutrient-dense foods, 32–34

O

obesity, 5–6

Ohsumi, Yoshinori, 17

onions

    Baked Chicken Breasts with Ginger Sauce, 152–153

    Basil Shrimp Ceviche, 190–191

    BBQ Chicken Flatbread, 122–123

    BBQ Meatballs, 114–115

    BBQ Meatloaf, 106–107

    Chicken Fried "Rice," 144–145

    Chicken Soup, 212–213

    Fried "Rice," 226–227

    Halibut with Ginger Sauce, 196–197

    Meatball Soup, 214–215

    Salmon Ceviche, 188–189

    Salmon in Ramen Broth, 206–207

    Salt-Crusted Fish, 182–183

    Shrimp Curry, 168–169

    Shrimp Fried "Rice," 180–181

    Slow Cooker Doro Wat, 156–157

    Slow Cooker Shredded Pork Loin, 94–95

    Thanksgiving Stuffing, 228–229

    Turkey Meatloaf with Dijon Sauce, 154–155

Orange Chicken recipe, 142–143

Orange Creamsicle Ice Pops recipe, 236–237

Orange Creamsicle Smoothie recipe, 88–89

orange drink mix

    Orange Marmalade, 262–263

Orange Marmalade recipe, 262–263

    Orange Chicken, 142–143

oxaloacetate, 30–31

oxidative priority, 25–26

P

parsley

    BBQ Chicken Flatbread, 122–123

    BBQ Meatballs, 114–115

    Boiled Crab Legs with Spicy Mustard Sauce, 166–167

    Broiled Cod with Tartar Sauce, 164–165

    Broiled Scallops, 200–201

    Chicken Soup, 212–213

    Chimichurri Sauce, 260–261

    Grilled Chicken Breasts with Carolina BBQ Sauce, 128

    Grilled Filet Mignons with Truffle Mustard Sauce, 100–101

    Mediterranean-Style Grilled Swordfish, 202–203

    Saltimbocca-Style Chicken Breasts, 140–141

    Shrimp and Grits, 160–161

    Slow Cooker Ranch Chicken, 120–121

    Sorrento Fish, 192–193

    Thanksgiving Stuffing, 228–229

    Tuna Salad Dutch Baby, 186–187

Peel-and-Eat Ginger-Lime Shrimp recipe, 194–195

The P:E Diet (Naiman), 42

plant superfoods, nutrients in, 32

Poached Chicken Breasts recipe, 129

Poached Lobster Tails recipe, 177

Popovers with Tuna Salad recipe, 162–163

pork

    Baked Pork Tenderloins, 96–97

    BBQ Pork Chops, 102–103

    Breakfast Patties, 62–63

    Garlic Thyme Pork Tenderloins, 112–113

    Grilled Pork Chops with Truffle Mustard Sauce, 116–117

    nutrients in, 33

    P/E ratio of, 46

    Pork Chops with Dijon Vinaigrette, 98–99

    Slow Cooker Shredded Pork Loin, 94–95

    Sweet and Sour Pork Chops, 110–111

Pork Chops with Dijon Vinaigrette recipe, 98–99

pork rinds

    Fried Soft-Shell Crab, 176

poultry, P/E ratio of, 43

protein

    about, 9

    oxidative priority and, 26

    quality of, 43–47

    requirements for building muscle, 34

protein powder

    Apple Dutch Baby, 70–71

    BBQ Chicken Flatbread, 122–123

    Cinnamon Protein-Sparing Bread, 270–271

Cinnamon Roll Waffles, 72–73

Classic Angel Food Cake, 246–247

Egg Salad Sandwiches, 216–217

Popovers with Tuna Salad, 162–163

Protein-Sparing Bread, 270–271

Protein-Sparing Pancakes, 66–67

Protein-Sparing Waffle Buns, 272–273

Savory Dutch Baby with Lox, 68–69

Strawberry Angel Food Cake, 246–247

Strawberry Protein Pops, 242

Strawberry Shake, 86–87

Tuna Salad Dutch Baby, 186–187

Vanilla Angel Food Cupcakes, 248–249

protein to energy ratio (P/E), 42

Protein-Sparing Bread recipe, 270–271

Bread Pudding, 252–253

Classic French Toast, 74–75

Ham Omelet, 56–57

Slow Cooker Doro Wat, 156–157

Thanksgiving Stuffing, 228–229

Tiramisu, 254–255

Turkey Sandwich, 218–219

protein-sparing modified fasting (PSMF)

about, 7, 22–23

calculating target macros, 40–41

doing it the wrong way, 39

how it works, 24–34

implementing, 40–49

Krebs cycle, 26–31

maximizing time with, 48–49

nutrient-dense foods, 32–34

oxidative priority, 25–26

protein to energy ratio (P/E), 42

quality of proteins, 43–47

thermic effect of food (TEF), 24

Protein-Sparing Pancakes recipe, 66–67

Breakfast Sammie, 64–65

Protein-Sparing Waffle Buns recipe, 272–273

R

red snapper

Salt-Crusted Fish, 182–183

rosemary

Saltimbocca-Style Chicken Breasts, 140–141

Thanksgiving Turkey Breast, 146–147

S

sage

Thanksgiving Stuffing, 228–229

Thanksgiving Turkey Breast, 146–147

salmon

nutrients in, 33

Salmon Ceviche, 188–189

Salmon in Ramen Broth, 206–207

Salmon Jerky, 224–225

Savory Dutch Baby with Lox, 68–69

Salmon Ceviche recipe, 188–189

Salmon in Ramen Broth recipe, 206–207

Salmon Jerky recipe, 224–225

salt, sleep and, 49

Salt-Crusted Fish recipe, 182–183

Saltimbocca-Style Chicken Breasts recipe, 140–141

sandwiches

Egg Salad Sandwiches, 216–217

Turkey Sandwich, 218–219

Savory Dutch Baby with Lox recipe, 68–69

scallops

Broiled Scallops, 200–201

sea bass

Salt-Crusted Fish, 182–183

seafood. See fish and seafood

seafood stock

Shrimp Scampi, 204–205

shallots

Poached Chicken Breasts, 129

shrimp

Adobo-Style Shrimp, 178–179

Basil Shrimp Ceviche, 190–191

Broiled Shrimp with Cilantro Lime Sauce, 174–175

Mexican-Inspired Shrimp Kabobs, 184–185

Peel-and-Eat Ginger-Lime Shrimp, 194–195

Shrimp and Grits, 160–161

Shrimp Curry, 168–169

Shrimp Fried "Rice," 180–181

Shrimp Scampi, 204–205

Surf and Turf with Carolina BBQ Sauce, 172–173

Shrimp and Grits recipe, 160–161

Shrimp Curry recipe, 168–169

Shrimp Fried "Rice" recipe, 180–181

Shrimp Scampi recipe, 204–205

sleep, PSMF and, 48–49

Slow Cooker Doro Wat recipe, 156–157

Slow Cooker Ranch Chicken recipe, 120–121

Slow Cooker Shredded Pork Loin recipe, 94–95

Smoked Chicken Breasts recipe, 124–125

smoked salmon

    Savory Dutch Baby with Lox, 68–69

Snow Cones recipe, 240

Sorrento Fish recipe, 192–193

Souffle Omelet with Ham and Chives recipe, 58–59

soups

    Chicken Soup, 212–213

    Egg Drop Soup, 210–211

    Meatball Soup, 214–215

Spicy BBQ Vinegar Sauce recipe, 264–265

starvation mode

    about, 35–36

    metabolic adaptation, 37–38

    miscalculation of caloric intake, 36

    PSMF the wrong way, 39

Steak and Eggs recipe, 60–61

strawberries

    Strawberry Shortcake, 250–251

Strawberry and Cream Ice Pops recipe, 243

Strawberry Angel Food Cake recipe, 246–247

    Strawberry Angel Food French Toast, 76–77

    Strawberry Shortcake, 250–251

Strawberry Angel Food French Toast recipe, 76–77

Strawberry Pavlova recipe, 232–233

Strawberry Protein Pops recipe, 242

Strawberry Shake recipe, 86–87

Strawberry Shortcake recipe, 250–251

sugar

    nutrients in, 14

    sleep and, 49

Surf and Turf with Carolina BBQ Sauce recipe, 172–173

Sweet and Sour Pork Chops recipe, 110–111

swordfish

    Mediterranean-Style Grilled Swordfish, 202–203

T

tamari

    Adobo-Style Shrimp, 178–179

    Asian-Inspired Stir-Fried Turkey, 136–137

    Asian-Style Meatballs, 108–109

    Baked Pork Tenderloins, 96–97

    Bourbon Chicken, 148–149

    Chicken Fried "Rice," 144–145

    Egg Drop Soup, 210–211

    Egg Foo Young, 130–131

    Fried "Rice," 226–227

    Orange Chicken, 142–143

    Salmon in Ramen Broth, 206–207

    Salmon Jerky, 224–225

    Shrimp Fried "Rice," 180–181

    Sweet and Sour Pork Chops, 110–111

    Venison Jerky, 222–223

target macros, calculating, 40–41

tarragon

    Thanksgiving Turkey Breast, 146–147

temperature, for sleeping, 49

Thanksgiving Stuffing recipe, 228–229

Thanksgiving Turkey Breast recipe, 146–147

thermic effect of food (TEF), 24

The 30-Day Ketogenic Cleanse (Emmerich), 40

thyme

    Chicken Soup, 212–213

    Garlic Thyme Pork Tenderloins, 112–113

    Meatball Soup, 214–215

    Poached Chicken Breasts, 129

    Pork Chops with Dijon Vinaigrette, 98–99

    Thanksgiving Turkey Breast, 146–147

Tiramisu recipe, 254–255

tomato paste

    Salmon in Ramen Broth, 206–207

tomato sauce

    BBQ Meatballs, 114–115

    BBQ Pork Chops, 102–103

    Bourbon Chicken, 148–149

    Grilled Chicken Breasts with Tomato Basil Sauce, 138–139

    Slow Cooker Shredded Pork Loin, 94–95

    Sorrento Fish, 192–193

    Spicy BBQ Vinegar Sauce, 264–265

    Sweet and Sour Pork Chops, 110–111

tricarboxylic acid cycle (TCA), 26–31

triglycerides, 20

trout

Salt-Crusted Fish, 182–183

Truffle Mustard Sauce recipe, 100–101

Grilled Pork Chops with Truffle Mustard Sauce, 116–117

truffles

Grilled Filet Mignons with Truffle Mustard Sauce, 100–101

tuna

Popovers with Tuna Salad, 162–163

Tuna Salad Dutch Baby, 186–187

Tuna Salad with Dijon Mustard, 170

Tuna Salad Dutch Baby recipe, 186–187

Tuna Salad with Dijon Mustard recipe, 170

turkey

Asian-Inspired Stir-Fried Turkey, 136–137

Buffalo Chicken Meatballs, 150–151

Chicken Fried "Rice," 144–145

Cool Ranch Chips and Dip, 220–221

Egg Foo Young, 130–131

Thanksgiving Stuffing, 228–229

Thanksgiving Turkey Breast, 146–147

Turkey Frittata, 54–55

Turkey Meatloaf with Dijon Sauce, 154–155

Turkey Sandwich, 218–219

Turkey Frittata recipe, 54–55

Turkey Meatloaf with Dijon Sauce recipe, 154–155

Turkey Sandwich recipe, 218–219

V

Vanilla Angel Food Cupcakes recipe, 248–249

Venison Jerky recipe, 222–223

Hamburger Patties with Mustard, 92–93

W

white fish

Broiled Cod with Tartar Sauce, 164–165

Sorrento Fish, 192–193

wild game, P/E ratio of, 44

Y

yellow mustard

BBQ Meatballs, 114–115

BBQ Meatloaf, 106–107

Carolina BBQ Sauce, 267

Egg Salad Sandwiches, 216–217

Hamburger Patties with Mustard, 92–93

Mayo, 269

Popovers with Tuna Salad, 162–163

Tuna Salad Dutch Baby, 186–187

Turkey Sandwich, 218–219

More from Maria Emmerich

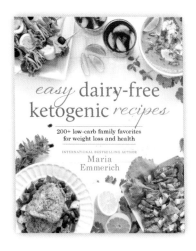

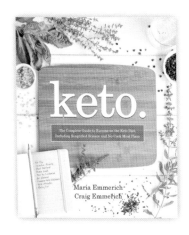

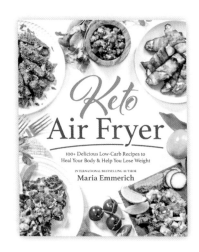

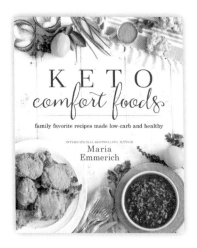

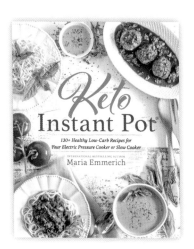

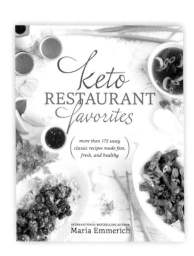

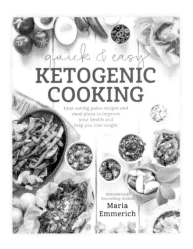

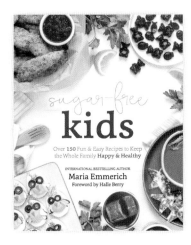

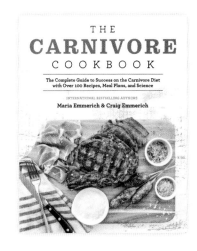

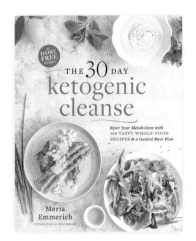

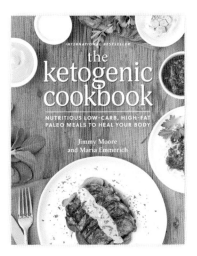

Find Maria's cooking videos on YouTube using this QR code!